Praise For *Steal*

"It is an absolutely necessary read for anyone who finds themselves at a junction in their lives where they know, without a doubt, that it's time to re-think their healthcare choices but have no clue how to proceed."

—J.D-B., wife and mom of two twenty-somethings, professional cellist

"I LOVED your book! Thank you for explaining why the medical field is where they are today, and why most insurance doesn't cover natural methods. It beautifully describes why holistic methods should be used along with medical, if needed."

—G.V., mother of seven, grandmother of nine, chiropractic patient of 50 years

"Stealth Health is a guide to be proactive about your health while shedding light to the issues of modern medicine and ways to control how you are influenced."

—D.A., PhD candidate with a concentration in Neurodegenerative Disorders and Fragile X Syndrome and, ironically, a lover of headbanging music

"Stealth Health presents the paths toward health as easy and understandable, in a time when it seems a large uncoated "pill" to swallow. Resources are out there to get answers and take your health into your own hands in an educated way."

—J.S., RN, seeks a better way along with her osteopathic doctor husband

*"It's a book that encourages you to tap into your innate
healing ability which we all routinely forget is there!"*

—S.K., massage therapist and CranioSacral therapist

*"Stealth Health challenges everything we think we know
about illness, while providing the questions we need to ask
to put the power of health choice back in our hands."*

—S.S., psychiatrist, entrepreneur, and
Tap the Potential business coach

*"Stealth Health is useful for someone who had no clue they could
even question conventional medicine. This book will enable the
reader to get further help if they want to make real changes in life."*

—C.D., mom of three, wife of an entrepreneur

"Stealth Health is the playbook to take control of your health."

—D.D, Profit First professional and proud dad

*"Stealth Health provides a step-by-step outline of
how to take over your health care future."*

—D.K., devoted wife of devoted husband,
manages her M.S. with alternative means

"As I was reading Stealth Health, I realized how many resources I have and don't use like I should, and the impact it has on my life. I absolutely loved this book... A MUST READ!"

—B.S., artist, realtor, a great example
to her two granddaughters

"We need to remember that old habits don't define us. I love how Dr. Nancy speaks the truth. Stealth Health is a great eye opener for the society."

—M.K., retired RN, aspiring author,
star of Chapter 8 *Stealth Health*

DR. NANCY TRIMBOLI

STEALTH HEALTH

TAKE BACK YOUR POWER AND UNRAVEL THE MYSTERY OF YOU

Copyright Notice

Stealth Health: Take Back Your Power and Unravel the Mystery of You
© 2020 by Nancy Trimboli, DC

ISBN 978-1-7344421-0-6 (print)
ISBN 978-1-7344421-1-3 (ebook)
ISBN 978-1-7344421-2-0 (audio)

*To my patients of the past, the present, and the future:
thank you for allowing me to be an instrument in your
healing journey. Your trust in me is truly humbling.*

*To my future friends who strive to find a better way, I'd like to thank
my readers in advance. You allow me to fulfill my life's purpose.*

Contents

Introduction

GARRETT IS A super cute second grader. Not shy, but the strong, silent type in an eight-year-old body. He's a patient of mine.

Garrett's mom brought him to me at the recommendation of a friend. Before the first appointment, out of earshot so as not to upset him, she explained that he had aggressive tendencies, an inability to focus, and if he didn't improve his reading scores, he would have to repeat the second grade. She had adopted Garrett when he was a baby. His birth mother was a distant relative and a known drug addict. He'd had a rough go of it.

When I met her, Garrett's mom had a hopeful expression on her face, but her body was tense, and she had a weary look in her eyes that I knew all too well. I'd seen it on the faces of my patients—too many patients. It's the look of someone hanging by a thread. Upon examination, I found subtle distortions in his cranial alignment.[1] The cranial bones never fuse together, even in adults. This allows subtle movement and a pumping action of cerebral spinal fluid for better nerve transmission.

We started his treatment plan and within two weeks Garrett was doing his homework happily. Prior to that, homework produced scowling looks, a fight with his parents, and the possibility of a physically violent outburst. Garrett started to enjoy school and was much more easy-going at home. His aggressive outbursts stopped. He became pleasurable to be around. With this change in demeanor, his parents decided the next step was to take him

---

1   Upledger Institute International, "CST FAQs," Accessed October 19, 2019. https://www.upledger.com/therapies/faq.php.

off his Attention Deficit Disorder (ADD) drug. That was an easy decision because it barely helped anyway. He graduated from the second grade.

The summertime school break disrupted Garrett's appointments at my office. At the start of the new school year, his mother brought him in again for treatment, as he was once again morose and resistant to do his homework. The engaging, smiling second grade graduate that I had come to know was replaced by the scowling, slouching one of our initial visits. After two appointments he regained his good mood and started quickly and easily completing his homework. By the second month in third grade, he surpassed his reading score of the previous year and in math ranked the highest in the entire third grade.

At his obligatory school physical exam, Garrett's mom told the pediatrician how great he was doing with chiropractic care, about the reading and math scores, and overall being happier.

The pediatrician offered: "There's still some other medications we could try…" Garrett's mom was stunned. Why was the pediatrician's only comment to propose medication when there was obvious success? Was she not paying attention? Where was her fascination for a discovery of a non-drug approach? Wouldn't she want to share this with other parents of ADD children? What could be her motivation for only thinking of drugs? Ignorance? Or, worse, could it be kickbacks?

This scenario is not unique. You know it. The compulsory medical doctor appointments. The medical professionals that don't seem to be listening. The long wait times for an appointment. The camping out in the waiting room. The dead-end treatment recommendations. The drug prescriptions when you don't want to take a drug; you want true healing. But where do you turn? Who will listen? Who has better options?

I'm here to tell you that there *are* better options. And, they are right outside your back door. Perhaps not literally, but certainly within the confines of the county, state or province where you live. I will help you to gain confidence in your choices as you search for healing. Your wellness journey and your health issues are unique. You yearn for a personalized path that supports you, not a generic one. Individual care is what you crave. Compassionate listening is what you need. Solid solutions will put your health issues behind you, or at the very least, control their effects on you without dangerous drugs or the unknown outcomes of surgery. This is what you now demand.

The world is spinning faster it seems. Our meal choices are decided by what is quicker or agreeable to the kids, rather than what is better. We wage chemical warfare on our hair follicles, on the weeds in our landscaping, and on the germs that cover surfaces in our homes. Our sleep is disrupted by blue screens, stress, and addiction to the current TV drama. We spend more and save less. Our time is filled with activity but no joy. Medical care has become mechanized. Big medical business groups now incorporate your small, local doctor's office into their conglomerate networks, changing how you interact with them.

You march and run and bike in charitable events promising to cure every disease on the planet. Millions of dollars are raised and spent on research. Yet people become sicker and at an ever younger age.

- Shingles was a disease relegated to only the severely immuno-compromised twenty-five years ago. Now, the Centers for Disease Control (CDC) estimate that one of three healthy adults will suffer from it at least once in their lifetime.[2] As distressing as that is, in 2002 a researcher predicted such a rise in shingles cases would occur with mass inoculation for chicken pox.[3]

- Chronic kidney disease rates are estimated to be 14% of the United States population and has remained steady since 2004.[4] In the last forty years since Medicare began paying for dialysis, kidney failure rates multiplied by a factor of forty-seven. Dialysis centers are now profitable business ventures collecting $34 billion yearly from Medicare alone.[5]

2   Centers for Disease Control and Prevention, "Shingles: Burdens and Trends," Accessed August 15, 2019. https://www.cdc.gov/shingles/surveillance.html.

3   Goldman, Gary, "The US Universal Varicella Vaccination Program: CDC Censorship of Adverse Public Health Consequences," *Annals of Clinical Pathology* 6, no. 2 (2018): 1133. https://www.jscimedcentral.com/Pathology/pathology-6-1133.pdf.

4   National Kidney and Urologic Diseases Information Clearinghouse, "Kidney Disease Statistics for the United States," Accessed September 15, 2019. https://www.niddk.nih.gov/health-information/health-statistics/kidney-disease.

5   Shinkman, Ron. "The Big Business of Dialysis Care," *NEJM Catalyst*. Accessed June 9,

- Male infertility has been on the rise over the last fifty years with speculation that the increased use of chemicals in our everyday world may be the cause.[6,7]

- Auto-immune disorders, a twentieth-century phenomenon, affect between twenty-five and fifty million Americans.[8] Treatments actually dampen immune function, potentially leaving the body vulnerable to infection and cancer.

How did we get here? Even more disturbing: how do we heal ourselves when the trend toward sickness is so strong? While Americans are exercising, cutting calories, and have a nearly endless amount of information at their fingertips, conventional medical providers have longer wait times and seem to listen less. To add to the frustration, the tools for healing in our medical system afford no healing at all. At best it masks the symptoms. Or manage the end stage of chronic disorders like heart disease, diabetes, back pain and the untreatable cancers. It's the norm to use drugs and intervention to suppress the symptoms of a disorder rather than solve the underlying issues. When pain meds don't work, then anxiety disorders are blamed for physical complaints.

The United States has the highest infant mortality rate compared to twelve other wealthy, industrialized nations.[9] That statistic has not changed or improved in twenty-five years. What are we missing? Where is the real healing? How could the miracle of life that brought us into the world not be able to keep us healthy?

2019. https://catalyst.nejm.org/the-big-business-of-dialysis-care/.

6   Carlsen, E., Giwercman, A., Keiding, N., Skakkebaek, N. E. "Evidence for Decreasing Quality of Semen during Past 50 Years," *British Medical Journal* 305 (1992):609. Accessed June 9, 2019. https://doi.org/10.1136/bmj.305.6854.609.

7   Mesnage, Robin and Antoniou, Michael N., "Facts and Fallacies in the Debate on Glyphosate Toxicity." *Frontiers in Public Health* 5 (2017) :316. Accessed June 9, 2019. https://doi.org/10.3389/fpubh.2017.00316.

8   Scleroderma News, "10 Facts and Statistics About Autoimmune Diseases." Accessed August 15, 2019. https://sclerodermanews.com/2017/10/30/autoimmune-facts-statistics/.

9   Gonzalez, Selena and Sawyer, Bradley, "How does infant mortality in the U.S. compare to other countries?" *Peterson-Kaiser Health System Tracker* (2017) Accessed June 9, 2019. https://www.healthsystemtracker.org/chart-collection/infant-mortality-u-s-compare-countries/#item-infant-mortality-higher-u-s-comparable-countries.

Not only is the world going faster, the world is becoming more expensive. Even with the Affordable Care Act of 2008, healthcare costs continue to rise.[10] Medical test costs are rising while drug prices have gone through the roof.[11,12,13] There seems to be no brakes on this runaway train of health expenses coupled with lackluster results.

Maybe we are searching in the wrong places. We've all been there. We've gone to our medical doctor looking for a miracle, and we are handed a prescription. What were we expecting? This is a medical doctor. That's what they do. They prescribe. They diagnose a disease and treat the disease with drugs and surgery. When someone tells me that they went to their medical doctor for a problem and they were disappointed when handed the white slip of paper, I wonder. I wonder what we search for that seems so elusive. Why do people continue to pursue conventional medicine in spite of the dead-ends and failures? I think I know the reason. We just give in. We are in the position of not knowing what to do or how to fix the problem. We continue to go back to our medical doctor because there is always hope that *this* time it will be different. That *this* time lightning will strike, and we will find the answer. Time and time again we are disappointed.

We are looking for a new way of thinking about health and healing.

Here's the news flash: Our bodies are not faulty, they are miracles. At the moment of conception, two half-cells unite to form one brand-new, never-before-seen cell that splits and divides and forms new cells. The cells continue to divide and differentiate until, nine months later, we have a baby. Two half-cells become 40 quadrillion cells in 280 days. Each cell has its own function and structure and it works perfectly. This is the miracle of life. The miracle does not escape us just because we are born. It is still within us.

---

10 Sherman, Erik, "U.S. Health Care Costs Skyrocketed to $3.65 Trillion in 2018," *Fortune*, February 21, 2019. Accessed August 15, 2019. https://fortune.com/2019/02/21/us-health-care-costs-2/.

11 Frakt, Austin, "Something Happened to U.S. Drug Costs in the 1990s," *The New York Times*, November 12, 2018. Accessed August 15, 2019. https://www.nytimes.com/2018/11/12/upshot/why-prescription-drug-spending-higher-in-the-us.html.

12 Robert, Langreth, "Drug Prices," *Bloomberg*, Updated February 5, 2019. Accessed August 15, 2019. https://www.bloomberg.com/quicktake/drug-prices.

13 Rosenthal, Elisabeth, *An American Sickness: How Healthcare Became Big Business and How You Can Take It Back* (New York: Penguin Books, 2018), 148.

How can your body be labeled as diseased, ill, or damaged when it is a miracle? Where is the healing?

The healing arts we hear of occasionally, like acupuncture or homeopathy, are rarely recommended by a medical doctor. The reasons for that are simple, basic, and fundamental. It's merely a different perspective, a different philosophy. Not a wrong or dangerous philosophy, just different. Because of that, most medical professionals don't understand it.

In my twenty-five years as a busy practitioner of chiropractic, I've seen over twenty thousand individual patients. They have consulted with me for everything from panic attacks to slipped discs to infertility and everything in between. My education consists of a bachelor's degree in biology, after which I earned my Doctorate in Chiropractic. As my mom used to say, I'm a smart cookie. I have an excellent reputation with local medical doctors, mostly because of an interaction with a fourteen-year-old patient when I was in practice for about two years. I spotted an abnormality in her walking that prompted me to send her immediately across the hall to the neurologist. She had a bone infection that required two weeks of intravenous antibiotics in the hospital. My referral may have saved her life or her leg. The news of my referral must have made it through the phone tree to all the medical doctors in my county. To this day I have patients say, "My doctor said not to see a chiropractor. Then I told them it was you. He said, 'Oh, okay, it's Nancy? That's fine, she's okay.'" The biggest fear of medical doctors for their patients related to holistic healing arts (like chiropractic) is that the practitioner will not refer a patient for crisis care when needed. Because I made that immediate referral, I quelled the fears of every medical professional, even now, twenty years later. The sad part? Any chiropractor would have done the same. We don't want patients who are in a crisis in our office. A large part of our professional training in chiropractic is teaching us when to make that referral. I am not unique in this regard.

The fact that conventional medicine is failing its patients is not the fault of the medical doctor. I have friends who have medical degrees and are in practice. For the most part, they truly want to help people. But I feel sorry for my medical doctor friends. I feel sorry that their toolbox is so limited, and potentially dangerous. The third leading cause of death in the United States is medical errors. Only heart disease and cancer top medical errors.

Some researchers say that the deaths due to medical errors are close to 440,000 Americans per year.[14] And, rarely does the death certificate list the error as the cause of death. Medical intervention is dangerous. Drugs have side effects. Individuals respond to drugs differently. The people administering the medications are human and can make human errors. Medical care is also necessary. We have extended our life expectancy by saving people from otherwise fatal accidents, injuries, and illnesses. Drugs and surgeries can save lives and improve function. But there must be a better way. And there is.

Over the last twenty-five years, I have assisted people by using the chiropractic adjustment. I have also assisted them on their paths to find true healing. Because my chosen profession is a healing art that is, by definition, outside of the drug prescribing arena, I am free to discover holistic remedies. I am not confined, like many of my medical doctor friends, to a predetermined mode of thinking. Thus, I have become a resource for many thousands of patients searching for alternative, holistic healing remedies. My mantra has been and will continue to be: My job is to figure you out, whether it is within my four walls or not. To this day I still recommend medical intervention when warranted. But my first mission to my patients is to find a better way if possible. A world of opportunity for health and healing is available, and very often right outside your back door, even in your own town. You just need to learn how to look for it.

You are on a health mission, or you want to be. If you've picked up this book, there is an underlying urge to find a new path, motivating change in your approach. Likely in your past there has been more than one dead-end. Day after day you suffer, putting on a smiling face for those that depend upon you. I commend you for continuing the search for true healing even though you are tired and in despair. Determination is driving you. Innately you know that healing is out there. Where exactly, you aren't sure.

When embarking on any mission, you need to ask yourself about the destination. Asking better questions will help. Some questions are defeating. Questions like "Why can't anyone help me?" and "What if I'm like this forever?"; these will get you nowhere. Asking better questions opens up the

---

14 Sipherd, Ray. "The third-leading cause of death in US most doctors don't want you to know about." *CNBC.com*. Accessed June 9, 2019. https://www.cnbc.com/2018/02/22/medical-errors-third-leading-cause-of-death-in-america.html.

possibility of better answers and allows you to be mentally available when the right person emerges with a new idea or a successful path for you to follow. In this book I will tell you the exact right questions to ask to illuminate innate insights and attract the people and ideas into your life that are needed. At times, the exact right thing for you will be a medical test, or medical treatment. I will help you to be the master of those decisions. You will know more about the testing and treatment, and your body, than even your medical professional. Your uniqueness is lost on conventional medicine. Medical professionals are taught to treat a named diagnosis, not you the individual. When you take back your power through knowledge of your own body, the medical professionals work for *you*. You direct your own healing journey.

The people who will become your allies in healing and their impactful ideas are all around you. Up until now, you haven't been able to see them or know about them. This is normal and common. Most of these techniques and people run contrary to the established norms. Some of them must adhere to the rules of the Food and Drug Administration or the Federal Trade Commission and therefore cannot be forthcoming with the benefits of their treatments or remedies. Your job is to sleuth out the information that has been purposefully hidden from you. Practitioners of certain healing arts may be restricted in your state due to archaic state laws. Although these people exist, you will never see a website or a telephone listing for them. As an example, in fifteen states, midwifery is unlicensed. A certified midwife would be at risk for criminal prosecution if she assisted in a labor and delivery. Even for me, if I was to advertise that patients of mine had gotten permanent relief and resolution from their anxiety, or their infertility, I would be slapped with disciplinary action from my own state board of chiropractic. We are all flying under the radar. As are you. Stealth Health is now the code word for your mission, Mission You.

If all these wonderful people who can help you with these remedies are not in plain view, how do you find them, you may be asking? Practitioners like us all stick together. We are allies that remain in the shadows. Those health providers that run counter to conventional medicine and drug therapy tend to know each other. I will teach you how to find reputable people that will be your allies on this journey. They will, in turn, share their wisdom and connections. You'll be able to tap into their contact list again and again. Because the trend of embracing holistic care is strengthening, that circle of resources is widening. You are on the precipice of the fall of The System that has worked against you your whole life, wreaking havoc on your health at the same time. You have perfect timing.

But I caution you that there are also channels of false information that may lead you astray. I have seen this time and again. Well-meaning people, like Garrett's pediatrician, or entities invested in distracting you, can lead you off your path of healing.

Who to Believe

Sarah, a longtime patient of mine, stopped drinking diet sodas and noticed a drastic reduction in her headaches. Until a coworker told her that she had seen on the evening news that NutraSweet was safe and approved by the Food and Drug Administration and the American Diabetic Association. A month later, Sarah was back in my office complaining of headaches. Her coworker had led her astray with false information. While those FDA and ADA approvals may be true, the connection between Sarah's headaches and diet soda was very real.

Mission You, should you choose to accept it, will not be a walk in the park. But you've been through the roughest part of it. Because of your health issue, you have felt the sadness of missing parts of your life. You've been in survival mode unable to enjoy the parts that bring you the most joy. The regret of not having the life you intended at this point can be crushing at times. You were *supposed* to be part of a great symbiotic relationship, being the attentive parent, or traveling the world. Pointless medical tests have left you frustrated and broke, and the lack of compassion of medical personnel is unimaginable at times. You have been trying your darndest. But you have fallen short. Do not fear. Help has arrived.

And, I know, your situation is different. Your problems are complex. Even so, there is still a path to healing for you. The magic of *true* healing is that it relies on the wisdom of the body. Your body is a walking, talking, breathing miracle. Self-healing and repair are what our body does best. But only if it has the basic building blocks, and the obstructions to healing are removed. That's what holistic care does. It removes the things blocking your path. Your body has 206 bones, over 600 muscles, and 40 quadrillion cells. Millions of neural synapses fire every second of every day. It all works —perfectly, unless it doesn't. You aren't *all* messed up, just some nuances are out of synch. I will show you how to regain order. I promise that by the end of this book, as you turn the last page, you will be well into Mission You. You will have garnered the energy to accept the mission. You will have the start of an arsenal of resources at the ready. These resources are there for you, willing and able to help. The community of professionals that are in your back pocket are fully invested in your health, healing and well-being. No more dead-end appointments or testing. No more dangerous drugs with questionable benefits. I promise that you will be confident in directing your own healing journey. A world of opportunity exists and it is waiting for you to discover it.

Chapter 1

MISSION YOU: YOUR FIRST STEPS

"Nancy, you really need to get a colonoscopy. I'll tell you where to go," Dr. Gupta says in his heavy Indian accent. "In the meantime, try this medication with raisin."

Raisin? I thought. I don't want to ask for clarification because I am already embarrassed beyond belief.

The gremlin that lives inside my gut starts making noises at about ten a.m. and sounds like it is moving furniture. It seems like the imaginary armoires, couches, and coffee tables will start on the right side of my belly and slowly move to the left. I haven't had a normal bowel movement in six weeks whereas before you could set a clock to me: seven a.m. every day.

Now, what I had *several* times a day, was a severe urgency to get to the bathroom, but no substantial solids emerge. The cramping and pain I have doubles me over, takes my breath away, and I need to stamp my foot fiercely to survive those ten long, miserable seconds. Luckily, my symptoms abate during my workday, except for the loud gurgles and clunks coming from my bowels. I'm sure my staff think I am dying. And my patients? I hope they can see that my care is valuable in spite of the fact that I obviously can't help myself based on the noise coming from my gut. I get into the habit of speaking louder or making a noise just at the moment the "furniture" would shift.

In our little cluster of suburbs outside Chicago, Dr. Gupta is the go-to general practitioner for all the doctors and nurses. He never charges me for consultations and is always full of fatherly admiration of my work with my patients. He treats every patient the same way, because everyone loves him. By the time I make it to his exam room, I am usually at the end of my rope. He's probably seen me cry more than any other human.

For my problem, I have already consulted two chiropractors. I have been taking probiotics every two hours for weeks, done an allergy elimination technique as it had previously proved beneficial, and have tried all the home remedies that I could think of. All with no help. I consider it could be due to stress. I do some meditation, write some affirmations. No help.

Dr. Gupta had written me this prescription and I fill it. Perhaps he had said resin, not raisin. Resin? Like tree sap? As in the sticky black tar I used on my bow in high school orchestra?

I knew this approach was a dead-end. I knew that I would decide against a colonoscopy, but I filled the prescription for this "raisin" medication mostly to keep taking steps toward the elusive endpoint of healing. It was as if I was thinking that a lightning bolt from the sky would, *shazam*, strike me and fix me.

I am sure you have been in a similar situation. Like me, you wish that could be the case: that lightning would strike. That one person would look at you and say, "Here it is! Here is the magic button that will make it all go away."

Chiropractic can be the instant cure in some cases, but those are few and far between. Chiropractic sees its share of overnight miracles, as do all the healing arts. For you and your problem right now, though, this is probably not one of those times. You may look for excuses for your problems. Such as, "my father had Irritable Bowel Disease, maybe that's what it is," or "my Aunt Gerta had migraines, it's probably hereditary," or "maybe I'm just getting old." I hate that last one. Most people never recover from believing that one.

You have been where I have been. I know it. You are in the dark. You can barely speak about your issue, or you speak of it too much. Those close to you are sick of hearing about it. They are so sick of it they begin to think you are just seeking attention. Or, that you are simply stressed from the kids, the job, the maintaining of the house, the taking care of everyone else. They tell you that it's all in your head. Take it easy, they say. Slow down. If you slept in, everything would be better. It's tough to hear these dismissive statements from the people who vowed to stand by you in sickness and health. The truth is, they may not know what to do with you anymore. They don't see the clues; not like you do. *You* know a good night's sleep isn't going to magically solve your problem. It's not all in your head. What you are experiencing is real.

Your Health is a Mystery to Unravel.

Day by day you know that there is more at stake here than just your symptoms. What's at stake is the vision you had for yourself at this time in your life. You would be enjoying life; you wouldn't be so fixated on this problem. All your ducks would be in a row. You wouldn't be so overwrought with this issue. This issue that won't go away.

Let me guess—you've had an army of professionals try to figure you out. This army has, to this point, if you really think about it, let you down. Up until recently you probably didn't think about it because you were just dealing with it: you were tolerating your symptoms and following orders. Until one day, you hear a little tidbit of a solution for your problem. And you ask yourself, "Why haven't I heard of this? Why didn't one of the army of professionals tell me to seek such a solution?" That's when you realize: Even they don't know the answer. Because they aren't looking for the answer. They are part of The System that pushes you through the steps, through the hoops, through the assembly line without regard for actual results. That's when you start to feel angry, abandoned as a human being.

Suddenly, you are aware of yourself on the assembly line as part of The System. It doesn't feel right, and you don't feel good. And so, you are handed Mission You. The mission was not apparent to you before. You were left in the dark by seemingly educated professionals that seemingly had answers. Not good answers, but answers. And these answers, as you think back, benefitted them, not you. You've put up with long wait times and possible side effects from medication you may not have needed. Your trust is wavering.

Here it is, your turning point. You have hit so many dead-ends that you are beyond disappointed, disenchanted, or discouraged. You are now determined. You know that this mission is yours to travel alone. Although you will encounter allies along the way, this is a solo mission and you must take the lead role. Your mission, if you choose to accept it, is Mission You.

Your determination is nearly palpable. Seeing into the future, you picture yourself free of your current issues. Life-changing decisions made with one goal in mind, with you as the priority, are ready to be made. All the other distractions of life can wait because when you solve the mystery of you, everything is better, easier. Life will be joyous again.

At this moment, you may not believe that you have the smarts for this. However, you do. All those big words used in medical care are learnable. I will teach you how to do that. Your body, magical though it may be, *is* understandable. It is not necessary for you to know everything about every organ, just to learn about *your* issues. The resources to understanding I will share with you. You may think that you've been told you have XYZ diagnosis, and the only thing you can do is stay on ABC drug indefinitely. You may have been told wrong. You may think that you lack the energy to even try to figure yourself out. You may think you have too many responsibilities, you are too tired, you have too many appointments for medical tests and office visits to even fit it into your schedule. I will impart to you a structure, and even a little motivation, to pursue Mission You. Your reward is no small trinket. To regain your life, to reclaim your dreams, and to be able to concentrate on the things that matter most—that is what awaits you.

Once you make the decision to take back your power, a shift will happen in you and in the world around you. Opportunities will open up. Information once hidden will become obvious. Helpful people will suddenly appear. I have done this for myself and I will teach you how to do it for yourself. I have been a guide for thousands over the last twenty-five years. I've seen people improve as they age, become increasingly active and full of life, rejecting the detrimental "usual and customary" routines that have made others sicker and sicker. The numbers of people like you, embracing a new way of thinking, are growing daily. A surge is rising. And all it takes is a shift in perspective.

Keep in mind that the world, as it is today, works against us. Forces with unknown agendas want to see you and me fail. The underlying motivation may be unclear, but now we are on to them. They might be watching us but now we know it. This is why we work undercover in Stealth Health mode.

The Medical System Was Not Built with Your Health in Mind

The System, as you will come to know it, was built bit by bit. It encompasses primarily the pharmaceutical industry, the conventional medical model, and chemical companies including food companies. The advertising industry and the media play powerful supporting roles, with research and academia along for the ride adding collateral damage. Health insurance companies and federal government agencies, who you might believe would support better and cheaper ways to deliver healthcare, appear to merely echo the chants of the major players. Each component exerts influence over the other and is also dependent upon the other. If one player were to leave the game, we might see the whole thing fall apart. Maybe one day that'll happen. Don't hold your breath. It may not happen in our lifetime.

You were born into The System. If you were born in the United States in the last seventy years, you had no choice in the matter. The System has had a hold of you since the moment of conception because of the choices made by your mom and dad. Your birth may have been by cesarean section to accommodate a doctor's vacation schedule. Your mother may not have known that she had the right to disagree and to be firm with her birthing choices. The influences over them directed the nutrition you received, likely in the form of little glass jars of mass-produced baby food. Your health was no longer seen as a God-given right, it was seen as an entity that could only be understood by a person deemed smart enough to comprehend it. And who usually wore a white lab coat. The medical professional. The inborn awareness you possessed as a small child which guided you to sleep, to awaken, to rest, to play, to eat is slowly distanced from you. The System does not want you to trust your instincts. If you are confident about your health and your well-being and make choices that are part of the natural order, what need would you have for The System?

The System removed your confidence. Your grandma's Old World ways of maintaining and regaining health were not to be trusted, even though she was as fit and robust as any human. Your parents, and therefore you, were taught that health concepts were beyond your grasp. Every sniffle, cough, and sneeze were indicators for your mother to keep you out of school for a visit to the friendly MD, most likely to receive the new wonder drug: antibiotics. And it worked. Antibiotics tended to shorten the life of that illness. For the moment, that is, until it resurfaced.

The System, like any great foe in a spy mystery, is all-knowing, has its hands in all your daily affairs, seemingly giving you, no, feeding to you only the options that will keep you marching along as a dependent servant entrained to its agenda. It works all around you without you even being aware. The information you believe as truth may have been skewed to support all the various components—the pharmaceutical industry, research and conventional medical care, the chemical/food companies, the media and the insurance companies. You will learn that the choices you perceive as being made independently by you in healthcare and food actually keep you under its control. Your medical doctor, probably without their consent or knowledge, was trained in the ways of this insidious institution, The System.

The System only works if everyone believes that it works. If details of failure surface that disprove an inherent treatment, the deaths and chronic illnesses created by that once "proven, usual, and customary" treatment are dismissed. The poor judgement that created that treatment is never one that is addressed. Without missing a beat, new treatments are suddenly regarded as safe when in reality it is just a matter of time before another tragedy might occur. If a whistleblower musters the courage to point out the deficiencies, they are discredited and shamed. The System protects itself while pontificating with high drama that it is there to protect you. Nothing could be further from the truth. No wonder you are messed up.

But don't misunderstand me. Your medical doctor *is* on your side. Most medical doctors studied medicine because they wanted to help people. Medical school admission is very difficult to attain and it takes many years of sacrifice to gain entry, complete the schooling, and survive residency. Along this path, most medical students encounter fatigue, nutritional deficiencies, sleep deprivation, and are peons in a profession where status and hierarchy determine success throughout a career. The neurosurgeons look down on the orthopedic surgeons who look down on the internists. Dealing with life-and-death situations, learning the accepted protocol for treatment prescriptions, all the while managing extreme mental stress means that when a simple answer is presented, it can be a welcome relief. Simple answers mean that this drug matches this diagnosis. This surgical procedure matches this problem. Don't go to a chiropractor. If you eat right you don't need a multivitamin. Vitamin E is dangerous. When life and death are in the balance, simple answers reduce the stress.

Health insurance companies, at their inception in the early 1900's, were nonprofit, and designed to protect the life savings of their patients in the event of catastrophic illness, and to protect the religious-based charitable entities that created them. As new technologies for disease management started to increase costs, for-profit insurance companies were born. In the 1970s and 1980s insurance companies became more like a big business and left the philanthropic, public-centered roots behind.[15] Each began to limit its risk by not accepting all patients and by tiering premiums. At the time, many insurance benefits provided 100% coverage and drugs were cheap. Vaccines and antibiotics cost little and, for the mom with the sniffly child, the antibiotics worked (in the moment). This combination contributed to the trend of moms taking their kids to the conventional doctor. The financial burden of paying for doctor visits was largely removed because insurance paid for it, as long as there was a diagnosis.

Everybody wins.

Another big win was aspirin. In its natural form, willow bark was used as early as Egyptian times (3000-1500 BC). It was the most widely purchased pain reliever in the 1950s. We no longer ask why we have pain … just take an aspirin. Specifically, we are told in the 1967 TV commercial that "Bayer works wonders."[16]

In the mid-1990s the FDA loosened the advertising restrictions for television and print ads under the guise of increasing the involvement of patients in their own healthcare. *Direct-to-consumer-advertising* (called DTCA) allowed manufacturers to advertise prescription drugs directly to you. Suddenly drug commercials and magazine ads had extensive lists of side effects, and you'd think any sane person would reject that drug outright. You know the ones I'm talking about. The overdubbed voice says some variation of, "Side effects could include insomnia, hair loss, suicidal thoughts and

---

15   Rosenthal, *An American Sickness*, 14-18.

16   "Bayer Aspirin (1967) - Classic TV Commercial." *YouTube*. Accessed July 18, 2019. https://www.youtube.com/watch?v=BESIxDaWJ44.

tendencies, new or worsening heart failure, sexual side effects, spontaneous diarrhea at cocktail parties, memory loss, dizziness, eye disorders...." Possibilities like that should send people screaming while running in the other direction, but that has not been the case.

Since that time, the increase in dollars spent annually for prescription drug DTCA has risen by $5 billion. *All* advertising for the pharmaceutical industry, from the pens on the sign-in sheet at your internist's office, to the sponsorship of the 5K fun run, to the online ads for the psoriasis medication that could get you infected with tuberculosis, is estimated to be $29.6 billion per year. (That's almost 30 billion, which is the number 30 with nine zeros after it, by the way. Spent every year.) This includes the $20.3 billion for "marketing to medical professionals."[17] No, your doctor wasn't left out of this. More than $20 billion a year is spent on them alone. Advertising to individual medical doctors looks different depending on their interests, stature, and motivation. It could come in the form of the daily in-office lunch catering for the medical staff, or via a paid speaking engagement at medical conferences where a doctor might discuss a specific medication, or attendance to educational seminars in exotic places.[18] These and other gifts are not intended to be enticements. Somehow it feels like it is.

That advertising expense for the pharmaceutical companies created by the loosened FDA restriction of the early 1990s has an effect on us and on our doctors. For every $1,000 dollars spent on DTCA, twenty-four new patients were put on medication.[19] That's a big bang for the buck. Not only did this benefit the drug companies' bottom line, but it also created business for their slick and creative marketers, and sold advertising time on our favorite television shows and on pages in our favorite magazines. As our attention was riveted on the glossy ads and bouncing smiling blobs, an idea was planted. We were being channeled onto a specific path, the pharmaceutical path, to supposedly assist in our health challenges. Other

17 Schwartz, Lisa and Woloshin, Steven. "Medical Marketing in the United States, 1997-2016," *JAMA*® 321(1) 2019: 80-96. doi:10.1001/jama.2018.19320.

18 Elliott, Carl. "The Drug Pushers." *The Atlantic.* Accessed July 18, 2019. https://www.theatlantic.com/magazine/archive/2006/04/the-drug-pushers/304714/.

19 Das,Roonita. "Are Direct-To-Consumer Ads For Drugs Doing More Harm Than Good?" *Forbes.* Accessed July 17, 2019. https://www.forbes.com/sites/reenitadas/2019/05/14/direct-to-consumer-drug-ads-are-they-doing-more-harm-than-good/#228e8a224dfc.

avenues with information about holistic practitioners were overshadowed by the distractions that multitudes of dollars will buy. Without attention being drawn to them, those safer and more effective options seemed to barely exist. If only acupuncture had $2 billion a month in promotional advertising, you would have three acupuncturists. You don't. But I would bet that you have at least three, if not thirty, assorted bottles of over-the-counter or prescription medications in your home.

It's not your fault or your doctor's fault. Everyone is just doing their job. The drug manufacturers have a product to make, and shareholders want their returns. The advertising agencies have bright minds at work doing their jobs to earn a living. The medical doctors believe that they are getting the best and newest information from the best sources: a keynote speaker at a medical convention or a friendly drug representative. They just want to help you with your pain and symptoms.

At around the same time, the food industry got ahold of us. In addition to societal changes in the US, better advertising tactics affected the quality of our food choices. Cute talking cartoons of kitchen accessories and booming handsome voices taught moms that making dinner with something from a box was not only easier, her family would enjoy it more. The reason they likely *did* enjoy it more is food additives heighten taste senses in the brain[20] – but also create an addiction to the additive. The kids would ask for it by name, especially after seeing the commercial on TV. Do you think it was by pure chance that the food industry created food items that were a greater expense for the consumer which created greater profit, and at the same time had an addictive quality? Over the decades we have moved further from whole foods. The food companies offer us what is cheapest to make and package, using government-subsidized corn syrup, bad fats, and processing. And, whether it is due to the advertising or the flavor enhancers, we gobble it up.

---

20 Simontacchi, Carol. *The Crazy Makers: How the Food Industry is Destroying Our Brains and Harming Our Children* (New York: Penguin Group, 2007), 102-106.

The System is a Cycle that Feeds Itself

The players in The System rely on each other to perpetuate it. It's a cycle that goes round and round. The food industry robs us of basic nutrition, which causes symptoms and disease, which leads people to seek the one who has been deemed the only person to make health recommendations, the medical doctor. The conventional medical system is the gatekeeper for the pharmaceutical industry as they are the only ones who can write prescriptions. The product of the pharmaceutical industry does not cure disease; it attempts to subdue symptoms of the person with the disease. Side effects of those drugs prescribed lead to other symptoms which necessitate the need for additional drugs. The conventional medical route is awarded "usual and customary" status by the insurance companies. Meanwhile drugless healing methods are deemed "investigational" and not a covered benefit. (The fact that these methods are safer, can have true and permanent healing with no side effects, and have been around longer than conventional medical care is apparently inconsequential.) Research labs, which are extremely expensive to operate, must petition for grants. A lab that proposes a study that can stay within the confines of the norm has a greater likelihood of being awarded money and thus ensure its continued existence. And, the pharmaceutical companies have the deep pockets of cash to support research that, in turn, supports them.

It's not your fault you were born into The System. But you will have to fight to get out of it. You will have to demand a better way. Forces bigger than you with unlimited resources are covertly, and surprisingly overtly, brainwashing you, those close to you, and your medical professionals. Because of this, Mission You must remain a secret. You must be undercover, stealthy. Not everyone sees the damage as it's being done by The System. Nor do they want to point the finger of blame. These are people that may be close to you and they are mentally invested in the messaging of the advertising and support of the media. Don't fault them for this. You recognize The System for what it is. You can't alter past decisions, you can't change other people, but you can certainly make positive choices for the future. Take back your power by asking better questions of yourself and your healthcare providers. Use conventional medical technology to your advantage. Medical testing can help discern clues. You can choose to use drugs for very specific reasons, not blindly for a lifestyle choice. Utilizing the best that conventional medicine has to offer combined with the true healing of holistic methods, you can begin to unravel the mystery of you.

Lies The System Tells Us

In any action movie, the good spy encounters villains along the way. And just like any great enemy, the facts are amended to justify controlling truth, whether it be the menacing superpower, a drug cartel, an overly protected, overly budgeted corporation with shaky ideals, or a government gone corrupt. Misinformation masquerades as truth.

Cashing in on Aspirin

The first large-scale study to show a possible link between aspirin and the prevention of a second heart attack was published in 1974.[21] The numbers were not statistically significant, meaning a direct cause-and-effect relationship could not be established. Regardless, aspirin companies saw a great surge in sales due to this research study. What was not known, or at least not openly discussed, was the side effect of stomach bleeding from the prescribed aspirin-a-day which almost completely negated the benefit of preventing the second heart attack.

Let's pretend for a moment that I'm an executive at Spherewell Pharmaceuticals, the owner of Major Aspirin company. I'm in my navy power suit. It's 1988. Disco is done and I'm not into grunge. A research study was published saying that an aspirin a day would reduce the chances of someone suffering a second heart attack by about 44%.[22] In actuality, 44%

21 Elwood, P.C. "A Randomized Controlled Trial of Acetyl Salicylic Acid in the Secondary Prevention of Mortality from Myocardial Infarction," *British Medical Journal* 1, (1974): 436-440. Accessed September 16, 2019. https://www.ncbi.nlm.nih.gov/pmc/articles/PMC1633246/pdf/brmedj02178-0046.pdf

22 Steering Committee of the Physicians' Health Study Research Group. "Final Report on the Aspirin Component of the Ongoing Physicians' Health Study," The New England Journal of Medicine 321 (1989): 129-135. Accessed April 14, 2019. DOI: 10.1056/NEJM198907203210301.

is not significant. If it were 44 *times* less likely, or even 4 times less likely, that would be something. But not 44%.

Even so, Major Aspirin has a lot of new competition and we need an edge. With this new research, I could improve the profit margin of our stock and make my shareholders happy.[23] I jump on it. I meet with my drug reps. These are the very attractive, very accommodating, very smart and flashy people I send to meet medical doctors to teach them about medications. The physicians get pens and mugs with Major Aspirin written on them, notepads, plus tons of free samples to give out. It's the only way most of these docs find out about new products and research. So much information comes out every month, they don't have time to review it. Every day is filled with seeing patients. They need help with knowing what to prescribe and they get that help from the people that make the drugs. It seems a bit self-serving. But that's the way the world works. And it's legal.

As a side note to myself, the research also stated there was a slight increase in stomach ulcers with the aspirin group. I'm sure that's nothing to worry about. No need to mention it.

Fast forward to the year 2000. We all survived Y2K but we may not all survive an aspirin a day. For some people, an aspirin may reduce the chance of a *second* heart attack and certain strokes because aspirin thins the blood. Thinning the blood also poses a serious and potentially deadly risk of stomach bleeding.[24] Your stomach may be bleeding whether you know it or not. Are physicians still recommending an aspirin day? Yes, even to those who have *not* had a previous heart attack.

Major Aspirin is still doing fine in spite of a 2018 Harvard Health Online newsletter that outlines recent studies pointing to, well, aspirin may be no help at all.[25] And, over the years, it may have hurt a bunch of people. Oh well. Maybe we won't advertise the "take an aspirin a day as directed

---

23 Feder, Barnaby. "Market Place: The Stock Impact of Aspirin Report." *New York Times*, January 28, 1988. Accessed July 20, 2019. https://www.nytimes.com/1988/01/28/business/market-place-the-stock-impact-of-aspirin-report.html.

24 WebMD, "Even Low Dose of Aspirin Can Cause Intestinal Bleeding." Accessed July 20, 2019. https://www.webmd.com/drug-medication/news/20001109/even-low-dose-of-aspirin-can-cause-intestinal-bleeding#1.

25 Harvard Heart Letter, "Rethinking low-dose aspirin." Accessed July 20, 2019. https://www.health.harvard.edu/heart-health/rethinking-low-dose-aspirin.

by your doctor" thing anymore. It seems to be a controversial subject. But what a windfall for my investors over the last half century.

The debate continues, and people, maybe even you, still take an aspirin a day. As recently as 2014 researchers urged the medical community to re-evaluate the use of daily aspirin because of the direct causal link with the deadly possibility of stomach bleeding. I could find no evidence of any aspirin company paying damages to its users. Interestingly, there was never a direct link found to support the use of an aspirin a day, but it was pushed on us anyway. However, direct evidence of an aspirin a day causing bleeding ulcers is there. That message is either ignored or diluted to our detriment. But it benefits whom? The System.

Five Years Too Late

The drug Vioxx was introduced in 1999 as an arthritis pain medication. It was allotted $160 million in advertising; twice what Nike spent that year.[26] Vioxx was no better than Celebrex which was currently on the market, if only for a few months. Vioxx was marketed on the premise that clinical trials proved that there were fewer stomach problems associated with it, as compared to Celebrex. After being on the market for 5 years it had brought Merck $2.5 billion[27] in annual sales. But there was a problem with Vioxx. Horribly, by 2004, it had caused at least 88,000 heart attacks in the United States. Two-thirds of those people reportedly died from the drug.[28] And,

26 Gellad, Ziad and Lyles, Kenneth, "Direct-to-Consumer Advertising of Pharmaceuti- cals." The American Journal of Medicine, 120, 6. (2007): 475-480. Accessed July 20, 2019. doi: 10.1016/j.amjmed.2006.09.030.

27 Associated Press on NBC News.com, "Merck's profit slammed by charge, Vioxx: With- drawal of arthritis drug, tax charge lead to big earnings decline." Accessed August 17, 2019. http://www.nbcnews.com/id/8656235/ns/business-us_business/t/mercks-profit-slammed- charge-vioxx/#.XViEaeNKiUk.

28 Maugh, Thomas H. II, "Banned Report on Vioxx Published." Los Angeles Times, January 5, 2005. Accessed August 17, 2019. https://www.latimes.com/archives/la-xpm-2005-jan- 25-sci-vioxx25-story.html.

this will really put a thorn in your craw, the executives of the company that manufactures it knew the dangers as early as the year 2000.[29]

(Remember the blood-thinning effects associated with daily aspirin use? By a different mechanism, regular use of these types of arthritis pain medications, COX-2 inhibitors, has a similar effect. In this case, the clots that form after the blood thins cause the heart attacks and strokes.[30])

The Food and Drug Administration (FDA) is responsible for approving drugs to be marketed to the general population. Clinical trials are research studies organized by the pharmaceutical companies that demonstrate safety by having actual humans take the medication, and prove that the drug is more effective than a sugar pill for a specific symptom.[31] The new drug does *not* need to show that it is better than an already existing one or a natural remedy.[32] Participants in the study are subject to approval for the drug testing with a "run-in period."[33] The run-in eliminates people who have an adverse reaction from the drug, or possibly no response at all. Once written, the final research study does not reflect these non-responders or those who experienced side effects early on. Also, the number of participants in the final drug testing is small relative to the numbers of people who take the drug after it is made available to the public. This, combined with the "run-in period," may yield results overestimating positive effects and underreporting negative effects. It's only when the drug hits the mass market that the real problems can show up.

29 Horton, Richard, "Vioxx, the implosion of Merck, and aftershocks at the FDA." *The Lancet*, 364 (2004): 1995-1996. Accessed September 16, 2019. DOI: https://doi.org/10.1016/S0140-6736(04)17523-5.

30 News Medical, "Why COX-2 Inhibitors such as Vioxx Can Cause Heart Attacks and Strokes," Accessed August 18, 2019. https://www.news-medical.net/news/2006/12/02/21158.aspx.

31 FDA, "Development & Approval Process | Drugs," Accessed August 17, 2019. https://www.fda.gov/drugs/development-approval-process-drugs.

32 Light, Donald, "New Prescription Drugs: A Major Health Risk With Few Offsetting Advantages," *Harvard University Edmond J. Safra Center for Ethics* (blog), June 27, 2014. Accessed July 20, 2019. https://ethics.harvard.edu/blog/new-prescription-drugs-major-health-risk-few-offsetting-advantages.

33 Pablos-Mendez, A., "Run-in Periods in Randomized Trials: Implications for the Application of Results in Clinical Practice," *JAMA* 279:3 (1998): 222-5. Accessed September 18, 2018. https://www.ncbi.nlm.nih.gov/m/pubmed/9438743.

Dr. David Graham was the FDA employee who pushed to get Vioxx withdrawn from the market. He was labeled the "whistleblower" regarding the Vioxx scandal and took big personal risks to follow through with his findings. Senior FDA officials attempted to discredit Dr. Graham and his work, smear his name, and intimidate him to keep him from testifying before Congress.

In a candid interview in 2012 with Mannette Loudon, the lead investigator for Gary Null, radio host, author and alternative medicine advocate, Dr. Graham explained how the FDA is unable to protect us from dangerous pharmaceuticals.[34] He said, "As currently configured, the FDA is not able to adequately protect the American public … when there are unsafe drugs, the FDA is very likely to err on the side of [the pharmaceutical] industry. Rarely will they keep a drug from being marketed or pull a drug off the market. A lot of this has to do with the standards that the FDA uses for safety.… The FDA assumes the drug is safe and now it's up to the company to prove that the drug isn't safe.… No incentive is in place for the companies to do things right. The clinical trials that are done are too small, and as a result it's very unusual to find a serious safety problem in these clinical trials. Safety flaws are discovered after the drug gets on the market."

Congress passed an act in 1992 that creates additional funding for the FDA to hire the physicians and scientists needed to ensure drugs could be approved to market at a greater pace. Problems inherent in quicker approvals are what may add to the possibility that severe adverse reactions appear after the drug is used by the general public. After release, it is being used by hundreds of thousands of people rather than a thousand specifically selected people.

Dr. Graham continues, "For [the pharmaceutical] industry, every day a drug is held up from being marketed, represents a loss of one to two million dollars of profit. The incentive is to review and approve the drugs as quickly as possible, and not stand in the way of profit-making. The FDA cooperates with that mandate."

---

34 "The FDA Exposed: An Interview with Dr. David Graham, the Vioxx® Whistleblower," *Life Extension Magazine*, October 2012. Accessed June 11, 2019. https://www.lifeextension. com/magazine/2012/10/the-fda-exposed-an-interview-with-dr-david-graham/page-02?p=1.

Imagine if one or two million dollars a day was dedicated to promoting true healthcare options. At this time in history, we can only imagine.

Nutritional Supplements

Most of us find it mind boggling to walk into the supplement aisle of our natural food store. The grand scale of options available is only exceeded by the fact that none of the vitamin containers have any explanation of what good it might do. Prior to the 1990s, you could look to the supplement bottle on the shelf of the health food store to understand what conditions would benefit from taking the supplement. That all changed in 1994 when the FDA waged war on nutritional supplements. During that time, nutritionists and health food store owners rallied their clients and customers to appeal to their legislators to fight the FDA from removing nutritional supplements from the shelves or to force vitamin suppliers to adhere to burdensome testing. The compromise was to remove any words from the product that would indicate its use. All this was under the guise of protecting the public.

On Mercola.com an article posted in 2012 states vitamin and mineral supplements accounted for zero deaths for the year 2010, according to the US National Poison Data Systems annual report.[35] Although now two decades old, a 1998 study published in the *Journal of the American Medical Association* estimated that 128,000 people per year were hospitalized for adverse drug reactions, of which 106,000 died.[36] The majority of these adverse reactions were properly prescribed, properly taken medication. So, let's look at this again. In 1994 war is waged on nutritional supplements which account for zero deaths. At nearly the same time, while knowing that over 100,000 people die each year from them, pharmaceutical drugs are left

---

35 Mercola.com, "Dietary Supplements: Over 60 Billion Doses a Year and Not One Death, But Still Not Safe?" Accessed July 20, 2019. https://articles.mercola.com/sites/articles/archive/2012/04/23/defend-your-right-to-access-safe-dietary-supplements.aspx.

36 Light, Donald, "Institutional Corruption of Pharmaceuticals and the Myths of Safe and Effective Drugs," *Journal of Law, Medicine & Ethics*, 14 no.3 (2013): 590-610. https://papers.ssrn.com/sol3/papers.cfm?abstract_id=2282014.

to scamper on their merry way. Is it my imagination, or is this illogical? As my mom said, I'm a pretty smart cookie, and this doesn't make sense to me.

Chiropractic Malpractice Cost

In 2016, a tragic death occurred. A thirty-four-year-old mother and model died suddenly from a stroke that involved a blockage in her carotid artery, the main artery that supplies the brain with blood. *People* magazine, in an article immediately after Katy May's death,[37] and in the article from *Self* magazine, point to the fact that Katy had visited her chiropractor.[38] The articles were quick to implicate that it was the chiropractic adjustment that killed her.

Without knowing Katy, I assume that she had prior success with her chiropractor. She began suffering with neck pain and headaches after a bad fall at a photoshoot. Even the *Self* magazine article points to the fact that falls involving head injuries may cause these types of strokes. Being very active on her social media platform, Katy made a post that she had immediately gone to the hospital after the fall and was cleared by them. She was told that she had a pinched nerve. In an interview on *The Dr. Oz Show*, Katy's family did not blame the chiropractor for her death, which was a surprise to many. Dr. Oz closed the conversation mentioning the fact that carotid artery injuries such as this, although rare, can occur in vibrant, young people. He further said that there is no reason to avoid chiropractic and that healthcare professionals of all types should be more vigilant of the signs of stroke.[39]

Katy's death is tragic. No one knows for sure the exact sequence of

---

37   Mazziotta, Julie, "Katie May's Ex Wants '7-Figure' Payout for Their Daughter from Chiropractor Who Caused Her Death," *People.com,* October 31,2016. Accessed September 7, 2019. https://people.com/bodies/katie-may-estate-seeking-seven-figure-settlement.

38   Lanquist, Lindsey, "Model Katie May's Family is Suing a Chiropractor for Wrongful Death," *Self,* June 17, 2017. Accessed September 7, 2019. https://www.self.com/story/katie-may-lawsuit.

39   Clum, Gerard, "How Katie May's unfortunate death impacts the chiropractic community," *Chiropractic Economics,* November 22, 2016. Accessed August 18, 2019. https://www.chiroeco.com/katie-may-chiropractic.

events. It is possible that the fall Katy sustained created the tear in the carotid artery. The style of adjustment Katy received may have helped to progress an already existing issue. Your thought may be that getting your neck cracked could be dangerous, even obviously dangerous. Is it really? And, is that all chiropractic is? The System wants you to believe chiropractic is one thing: neck cracking and back cracking. Mobilization of the neck with the associated pop sound is just one technique in chiropractic; there are actually dozens of techniques and many have pressure lighter than your standard relaxation massage, with no popping. Check out the New Patient page of the website of my practice, Trimboli Chiropractic, at *www. TrimboliChiro.net*. I illustrate through video the low-force, no-popping techniques that I use.

So, is chiropractic safe? How can we know once and for all? Let's look at the facts. The facts that are based on numbers. Numbers created by actuaries. Actuaries work for insurance companies to calculate the real risk associated with, for example, the life expectancy of a person applying for a life insurance policy, or the risk of loss in the case of homeowner's insurance, or the risk of a profession, in this case malpractice insurance. Medical malpractice insurance prices are set based on the risk of each profession. In the medical profession, obstetricians pay $85,000 - $200,000 per year, every year, for malpractice coverage. Neurosurgeons pay $50,000 – $150,000, while the expense for an internal medicine doctor is $35,000.[40] Chiropractors pay $1,500 per year. No, there are no missing zeros. It's not *one hundred and fifty* thousand, it's *one* thousand five hundred. Your general practitioner pays 23 *times* the money per year for his malpractice insurance. Your obstetrician pays over 100 *times* more per year. That is an overt testament to the safety of chiropractic care. My eighteen-year-old nephew pays more for car insurance than I pay for malpractice insurance. If you saw him drive, you would agree that's fair.

---

40 Nabity, Colin, "How Much Does Medical Malpractice Insurance Cost in 2019?" *Leverage Rx* (blog). May 14, 2018. Accessed August 18, 2019. https://www.leveragerx.com/blog/medical-malpractice-insurance-cost.

Lowering Cholesterol as Big Business

While you may not be aware of the above lies, The System tells us one lie that has become accepted by most Americans as truth—that lowering your cholesterol is imperative for your health.

Cholesterol, in all of its forms, is an important part of every cell in our body. A coating called the cell membrane consists of fats, including cholesterol. The fats form a barrier between the inside and the outside world of each cell. Eat bad fats or artificially decrease the amount of fats in your body and you build weak cells.

Cholesterol is also the building block of hormones, the tiny messengers of our body that make all our basic biologic functions work. Our sleep, our sexual vitality and attraction, our moods, our energy level—the basics. Cholesterol also coats the nerves and is called myelin. If the myelin starts to wear away, the electrical firing of our nerves becomes faulty. This could, theoretically, cause physical disability, decreases in sensation, and impaired cognitive ability.

The war on cholesterol started in the late 1940s and early 1950s with the increase in heart disease deaths of WWII veterans. [41] Today, over 35 million Americans take statin drugs. In 1998 the new normal for blood cholesterol level was dropped from 240 to 200. If you had normal blood lipid level five years prior and were healthy, now, with the same blood lipid level, you are not healthy. [42]

Reports are mixed as to whether artificially lowering cholesterol reduces the chances of death of a heart attack or not. What if lowering the cholesterol artificially was a bad thing? Imagine that by reducing the needed cholesterol in your body, your basic human functions were diminished. Your drive to achieve, your happiness, your ability to sleep are dependent upon your body's ability to make hormones: testosterone in both males and females, serotonin and dopamine, melatonin, and all the rest. If those basic functions, the love of life, feelings of liberty, and the pursuit of happiness

---

41 Smith, Justin, Statin Nation: *The Ill-Founded War on Cholesterol, What Really Causes Heart Disease, and the Truth About the Most Overprescribed Drugs in the World* (Canada: Chelsea Green Publishing, 2017), audio version.

42 Welch, Gilbert, Lisa Schwartz, and Steven Woloshin, *Over-diagnosed: Making People Sick in the Pursuit of Health* (Boston: Beacon Press Books, 2017), 20-21.

were curtailed, what might you demand? Probably nothing. You're just too tired to argue. Think about this one... If the fatty myelin surrounding your gray matter (the thinking part) of your brain was reduced and your intellect were diminished, how much fight would you have for bucking The System? Not a lot, is my thought. I could be going out a limb here, but...is The System purposefully depleting us of our normal human urges in order to keep us contained, blindly following nonsensical directives? Are you becoming angry yet?

The New Reality

In Elizabeth Rosenthal's book, *American Sickness: How Healthcare Became Big Business and How You Can Take It Back*, she describes a perspective of medicine that is based on treatment and testing, with little concern for real patient outcomes. I believe that The System does not heal people; it creates patients. Documenting patient encounters with medical professionals has greater importance than the encounter itself. The family doctor that you grew up with, who maybe even made house calls, and watched you play JV soccer, is a rare thing today. Treatment options can be more frightening than the disease or condition itself. You, as the patient, have little to no control over costs of your doctor's visit, medications, testing or procedures. The referral maze of sending you from one doctor to another, all without any semblance of the concept to restore your health, leaves you with less money in your pocket and less time to do the things you enjoy. All your worst inner thoughts about conventional medicine and how it has changed in the last few years are founded. It is not your imagination.

Your first step on this journey is to recognize that this is the new reality. No longer is medicine a healing art. The conventional medical model has been degraded to an algorithm. For those of you who were out sick that day in high school when they mentioned algorithms, I'll explain. It is a series of steps from a problem to a solution. Different paths create choices along the way depending on the answers to the question in the algorithm. I'll include a simple version below. [43]

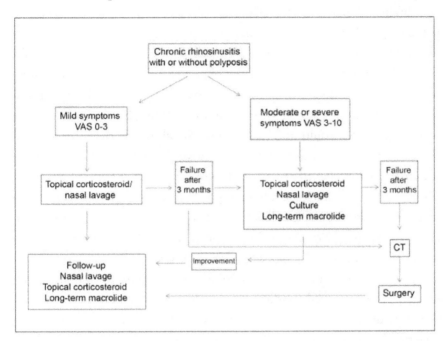

Key:

VAS: visual analog scale

CT: Computed Tomography

43 "Brazilian Guidelines on Rhinosinusitis," *Rev. Bras. Otorrinolaringol.* 74, n.2 (2008) pp.6-59. doi.org/10.1590/S0034-72992008000700002.

Start at the top box. Notice the Latin terms designed to put a crowbar in your brain and make you stop all searches for answers. *Chronic rhinosinusitis* is the diagnosis for which you may have been labeled. For now, let's not worry about the *with or without polyposis*. To untangle the meaning of a diagnosis, start shaving parts off the phrase and decipher each. Chronic, by definition, means the symptom has lasted a long time, which you find by doing an internet search for its definition. Rhino, if you were to search word origin, you would find means nose. We all pretty much understand sinus as related to our nose, but if you carve that word root off and do a search, you'll discover that a sinus refers to any cavity or space in the body. Okay, great. Store that little tidbit away for later use. The last portion of the diagnosis is *-itis*. Boy, is that label thrown around a lot. *Bursitis, tendonitis, plantar fasciitis, cystitis* are just a few of many. Looking it up tells you it means inflammation. *Inflammation.* That's a hot topic in the health news lately. What does it mean though? Doing a quick definition search will tell us that it is a "localized condition in which part of the body becomes reddened, swollen, hot and often painful, especially as a reaction to injury or infection."[44] So basically, the diagnosis says that your nose is stuffy because, well, it's inflamed, meaning swollen and painful. And it has been for a long time. Due to an injury (not likely), or an infection. (But why is an infection present?) Really, honestly, that's not much help. If a movie of your interaction with the conventional medical provider was spoken in Latin with English subtitles, the actor playing you would have said, "My nose is *stuffy*, my face *hurts*, and it's been that way *for a long time.*" And the actor portraying your doctor replied, "Ahhhh, in that case, with all the information you have shared, I am diagnosing you with LongTimeNoseCavityStuffiness. Let us commence treatment!"

No matter how silly that sounds, once a diagnosis has been established, the algorithm directs the recommended options, not your doctor. From the top box of the above algorithm labeled *Chronic rhinosinusitis with or without polyposis* follow the arrow to the right. In that box you will see VAS. The visual analogue scale, or VAS, is a way to communicate the level of pain

44 Lexico contributors. "Inflammation." In *Lexico.com*. Accessed August 18, 2019. https://www.lexico.com/en/definition/inflammation.

you are experiencing. If you have been to any type of health practitioner in the last ten years, you've been annoyed by being asked to assign a number to your pain. Simply, it refers to *how much does your symptom distract you from your daily activities?* If not at all, or you can ignore it, that's a zero to a three score. If you are mildly to moderately distracted by the discomfort but can still do all your activities in a normal fashion, that's a four, five or six. If there are one or more things that you cannot do at all, or in a normal fashion, that's a seven, eight, nine, or ten. Ten means you are unable to do much of your daily routine. (There are multiple types of pain scales other than the VAS. Pain scales used in trauma situations would be different.)

Suppose you were the patient that said, "Doc, I can hardly concentrate or sleep because my sinus pain is so bad." Your VAS score would likely be in the 5-6-7 range. Because the box to the right says *VAS 3-10*, follow the next arrow straight down to *Culture, Topical Corticosteroid, Long-Term Macrolide, Nasal Lavage* This tells us a few things. First, your medical professional will proceed with swabbing the inside of your nose and sending it to the lab to see if you have any unusual bacteria growing, that's the *culture.* Second, a prescription is written for two things: *topical corticosteroid and long-term macrolide.* It sounds mysterious but a quick search of word meaning tells you it's a cortisone cream to rub on your face, and antibiotics that you'll take for three months. Third, a recommendation is made for you to use a nasal irrigation device. This last one is probably the best advice from the entire algorithm.

Continue following the cascade of events to the next arrow and you see that we have a choice. Let's take the path the goes downward and turns left. *Improvement.* If you've improved, stay with me, keep following the arrow further left, a follow up visit will result in additional antibiotics, continued lavage, and you are sent on your way. At no point in the algorithm is the question asked about **Why?** inflammation or infection exists. Is there a food allergy? Is there an impedance to immune function or nerve transmission? Is there exposure to mold ? Also, there's no place for things you may have discovered that are helpful to your sinus problems. Things like supplements are not mentioned, for instance. Vitamin C[45] can be helpful for

---

45 Dhanawat, GS, "Rhinitis, Sinusitis and Ocular Disease – 2100. New approach to Treat Allergic rhinitis with Vitamin E, cod liver oil, and Vitamin C with use of

sinus congestion. Essential oils[46] can help you breathe easier. Chiropractic adjustments have been known to help some people with congestion.[47] But, nope, not there. Nor are homeopathic remedies[48] or lymphatic drainage massage[49] part of the plan.

Let's suppose, on the other hand, that you were *not* improved. Follow the arrow that goes right to *Failure after 3 months*. This means that for three months you've taken antibiotics (much to the detriment of your gut), used the nasal irrigation, and rubbed the cream on your face. Ninety days without improvement. The next arrow of the algorithm points down to *CT*. (Computerized Tomography is a 3D x-ray of the sinuses. You won't be tested on that. Just know that it's a medical test designed to find abnormalities in the bone or cavity. Radiation-wise it's the equivalent of about 200 x-rays.) This is a test that would look for something out of the ordinary in the sinuses. Which, if you have had this amount of sinus inflammation and infection for over three months, there will most definitely be something out of the ordinary. Likely there will be polyposis, aka polyps, (I told you we would get back to that later) which occurs because of prolonged irritation to the thin lining of your nose and sinuses. The blowing, sniffling, and constant excess liquid, aka swelling, underneath this delicate skin causes the lining to buckle. What will the CT show? Likely it will note pockets of infection and polyps. Which leads us along the last arrow to: *Surgery*. Surgery is not what you had intended when looking for help. Now that you've been traveling this road, the next stop is to make room in your busy schedule

Nasal Steroidal Spray," World Allergy Organization Journal, 6 no. 1 (2013): 175 doi: 10.1186/1939-4551-6-S1-P175.

46   Burgess, Lana. "Top 7 essential oils for sinus congestion," *Medical News Today*. Last modified February 27, 2019. Accessed August 18, 2019. https://www.medicalnewstoday.com/articles/324570.php.

47   Méndez-Sánchez R "Effects of manual therapy on craniofacial pain in patients with chronic rhinosinusitis: a case series." *Journal of Manipulative and Physiological Therapeutics* 35, no.1 (2012): 64-72. Accessed August 18, 2019. doi: 10.1016/j.jmpt.2011.09.012.

48   Zabolotnyi DI, "Efficacy of a complex homeopathic medication (Sinfrontal) in patients with acute maxillary sinusitis: a prospective, randomized, double-blind, placebo-controlled, multicenter clinical trial," *Explore: the Journal of Science and Healing 3*, no.2 (2007): 98-109. Accessed August 18, 2019. https://www.ncbi.nlm.nih.gov/pubmed/17362845.

49   Kecskes, Alex. "Lymphatic Drainage and Facial Massage can Help Sinus Infections and Allergies," *Pacific College of Oriental Medicine* (blog). Accessed August 18, 2019.

for the surgery date, recovery time, and pulling long sheets of blood and pus stained cotton out of your nose. Ugh. And does this really address the underlying weakness that caused the sinus issues in the first place? Will your sinuses now be perfect because you underwent the surgery? What are your thoughts? I'll let you answer; I think you're gaining the savviness to know.

Conventional medicine, almost no matter where you go, follows the same algorithms. A diagnosis leads to drugs, testing, and possible surgery. Other options are not in the picture, literally. The reason? *Evidence-based medicine.* This is a term used to describe current patient care guidelines. It is concepts based on peer-reviewed published articles in medical literature combined with "simple rules of science and common sense."[50] The peer-reviewed published articles draw conclusions from the results of randomized clinical trials (RCT for short). I know, all these hyphenated phrases and anacronyms make my head hurt too. Stay with me. In holistic care, like chiropractic, CranioSacral therapy, or prolotherapy, RCTs are hard to come by. That's because in this style of research study there are specific requirements. For one, there needs to be a "control" group. This is a segment of the people in the study who get a sham procedure or fake medication. In a drug trial some people get a sugar pill instead of the real drug. In that way the drug effect can be separated from the placebo effect.

The placebo effect means that you feel better because, well...no one knows why. Maybe it's because someone is paying attention, or it's the power of the mind believing you are being helped. The placebo effect can be dramatic and deserves additional study. For the sake of research studies, RCT's, the treatment needs to be shown to be not vastly, but merely slightly, more powerful than placebo.

Try to imagine doing an RCT on the effectiveness of acupuncture with a control group. You would have to think of a way to stick people with acupuncture needles in such a way as to not hit an acupuncture point. That would be your control group. It could be done, but not easily. It's the same for chiropractic. As soon as a chiropractor touches you, even to determine what spinal segment needs to be adjusted, the body responds.

50 Farlex contributors. "Evidence-based Medicine." In *The Free Dictionary by Farlex.* Accessed September 20, 2019. https://medical-dictionary.thefreedictionary.com/ evidence-based+medicine.

In either instance, the response may not be ideal, but it is still a response. It's different than having someone take a sugar pill. Holistic care models cannot be researched in the same way as drugs because a true control group is nearly impossible. Compared to medical applications, there is little data and few randomized clinical trials to support holistic care methods. These exist but are small in number and test the outcomes of a few people instead of thousands.

Masses of the population rely on their holistic care providers to help them make healing changes. Their testimonials, no matter how compelling, are considered clinical observations, not a randomized group. Meaning that no matter how much you love your chiropractor, no matter how much he or she has helped you, it is not a randomized clinical controlled trial. That coupled with other factors that favor the *status quo* leads to little to no mention in the conventional medical care algorithm for alternates. Hypertherm cocoons, tuning fork therapy, chiropractic care, matrix repatterning, or whatever alternative methods work for you do not find their way into the literature.

If You Can Spell Acetaminophen, You Will Solve Mission You

Conventional medical care does not care for the individual. I don't mean that your medical doctor doesn't care about your well-being. I mean that conventional medical care depends on creating a diagnosis and then treats that diagnosis using an algorithm. The diagnosis is achieved through medical testing or by default. By default, if no test comes up with an answer, you are given the diagnosis which most closely translates into a Latin term for your symptoms. If you go to your medical doctor for stomach pain, and no tests produce any origin for the pain, you will be labeled with a diagnosis of *gastritis*.

There's that *-itis* again. Let's break it down. We already know the word root *-itis* means inflammation, due to injury or infection, with pain and swelling. Searching the word root *-gast* (actually *-gastro*), tells us it indicates the stomach. So, after two thousand dollars' worth of testing and a lot of discomfort, you've just been told you have stomach pain. I'd say, "Eureka! Thank goodness. We figured that out." But that would be sarcastic. Suffice to say, there's no new information with this diagnosis. It didn't take a litany of tests to tell you that your stomach hurt.

You can see that it's been a no-win battle all along. The lies, the meaningless translations of your illness, the lack of interest in a better way. No matter how many dead-ends you have tolerated up to this point, you can take a new direction today. Accept Mission You and progress along a path to complete wellness. You can take the steps even if you have not taken any steps before. Today is a new day. A new day to make new decisions. A surgery date may be looming on the calendar, or you could currently be on multiple medications. You may believe that you have exhausted all of your resources, like I once believed.

This may sound daunting, but as you will see as we embark on this mission, Latin will become your second language. In order to speak with some of the sages of information on this mission, you needn't become fluent in Latin, just conversational. I promise you can do it. I also promise that you will become an expert in human biology. Your biology. Because conventional medicine treats a diagnosis, and not you as an individual, you will become your own human biology expert. No need to worry. You may not be able to recall the definitions of xylem and phloem from your seventh-grade science class, but I can guess that you not only know how to spell the word *acetaminophen,* you know how to say it. That means you can learn anything. The knowledge gained during Mission You is so extremely personal, it will become easy to understand. The strategies to fix your body will be devised by you and will prove to be effective quickly.

A world of opportunity for health and healing is right outside your back door. Perhaps not literally, but at least figuratively. You just need to ask the right people to help you access it. Our bodies are miracles that have amazing regenerative powers. We have been tricked by The System to believe that healing can only come from a pill or a potion, meaning something outside of ourselves. Advertisers want us to believe that if you have the right medication everything will be sunshine and rainbows. We know differently. We know that healing comes from within. All we need is to remove the interferences and allow change. Give the body what it needs, and it can make healing changes.

Your best ally may turn out to be your medical doctor or other medical professional. At times though, you will discover that you don't know whom to trust. You may find that your best advisor will seem to have suddenly switched sides. Not because they changed, but because you did. You will become more enlightened. You quite possibly will become more enlightened than your friends in healthcare. What is certain is that you will become a highly skilled undercover agent, a Stealth Health operative. Unless you really search out alternative health practitioners, they mostly remain unseen. When I first moved to Indiana, I was amazed at the variety of holistic healthcare practitioners in my area. You could do a course on Holosync® meditation, or experience an acupuncture session by a highly trained Chinese medicine doctor. Available then, and still available now is an Energy Medicine practitioner. Reiki wasn't on every street corner but nearly so. Therapeutic Touch was done by RN's in local hospitals. Cranio-Sacral therapy, Myofascial Release, and Rolfing® were in the next town. A local MD was shut down by the feds for doing chelation therapy on cancer patients. Off-the-grid homeopaths and colonic therapists work from their basements on the other side of the state line. And this is *Indiana*, middle America. I can only imagine what is available on the coasts.

My visit to Dr. Gupta was my last attempt, a flying leap to catch the helicopter rail as it flew away from me on the precipice. I was desperate to stop the downward spiral of helplessness into the dark answerless void. I was fresh out of my own answers and thought, as you may have, "Okay, alright, I'll just go to the *real* doctor. He'll have an answer." I feel deep gratitude that he tried to help me, albeit with his limited tools of "raisin" medication and colonoscopy.

My belief was that I was helpless and without answers, but it was not true. I *could* help myself. The answers were waiting for me to start the search. Starting the search, and accepting the path was all up to me. I would have to be my own best expert.

Even though I thought I knew all about human healthcare when I started my journey, I had zero understanding, and now after ultimately winning the war, am an expert on my problem. In my daily work as a healthcare provider, I have had the chance to coach others with this same issue, using the strategies that I learned to heal myself. Compared to everyone else, I was nearly my biggest challenge. To prevent a repeat of that experience, I continue to expand my knowledge today.

Most of your mysteries can be solved too. No matter what your background, your genetics, your past failures, or how little you think you know about your body, you can become the expert. Ask the right questions, find tidbits of life-changing information, and follow the paths that emerge. It takes some trust in yourself, I know. It takes some gumption to think that you can find the healing answers for yourself. That gumption is only matched by your determination created by the frustration you've been feeling for so long. You can do this. The answers are out there and waiting for you to accept Mission You.

As for me, I'm back on schedule, seven a.m. every day.

Mission You: Take Action

- Write your key motivators. Let's suppose I sprinkle magic fairy dust on you tonight. When you wake up tomorrow with Mission You implemented feeling improvements in your well-being, how will your world be changed?

Take a moment right now, I mean right now, and jot down the things that will be different about your life as you get better. These are your key motivators:

- Home life
- Family/ friends/ significant other
- Financial
- Professional
- Recreation / Artistic / Athletic
- Spiritual

Want more help with this? A free workbook is available from the downloads tab at www.DrNancyTrimboli.com. Print the *My Key Motivators* workbook page to organize your thoughts.

- With the key motivators you wrote, do one of the following:

  - Record yourself reading the list. Listen to the recording every day. Listening to your own voice speaking your own intentions will give your subconscious the job of creating that reality.

  - Post a note on your bathroom mirror with the one or two most motivating items.

  - Or, create a vision board collage by gluing clipped images and words from magazines onto poster board.

- This last step is important. I want to offer support. I can guess what's important to you but I would rather *know*. Go to our *Trimboli Insiders Group* on Facebook and post your top motivator. (Not a member yet? You'll find a clue at the end of Chapter 3.) Post a video if you are feeling bold. I want to hear your key motivating factors, the life that you are willing to fight for, the mission you are willing to put ahead of all your other priorities. You will find a community of like-minded individuals who have their own circle of resources. Allies come from unexpected places. As we share, we will shed the shackles of The System.

Chapter 2
TAKE CHARGE OF YOUR HEALTH

ETHAN HAWKE, THE character of *Mission Impossible* fame, picks up the receiver at a random phone booth in the Soviet Union. Or he puts on sunglasses that are inside a mini missile that has been shot to him while standing on top of a towering precipice in Monument Valley. A recording starts. The ultimate goal of the mission is laid out. It is sparse on details.

When Ethan Hawke is handed a mission, he never looks back. He doesn't question the mission, and he always chooses to accept it. Very few details are known at the onset. He may not know how events will unfold. Pertinent people will reveal themselves along the way. Creative ways to procure the needed intel to solve the mystery continually roil in his head. Information that at first seems random will eventually reveal its relevance.

When he accepts the mission, there is no second guessing. Never do you see him whining about what he could have done differently in the past. He doesn't look for the easy way out. Common sense keeps him safe. Savviness is more important than smarts, meaning that he can learn a few Russian words to decipher simple meanings, but having the ability to make good judgement has greater value.

There is no 'normal' protocol. If the normal, or conventional, route had achieved results, he would not have a job to do, a mission to complete. He has a trusted, small team that he can depend upon to have his best interest at heart. The other players that emerge along the way may confirm their allegiance, or they may disappoint him. He must act stealthily and be wary.

The villain is always out there with its own vested interests trying to foil his progress.

Being undercover means that Ethan is always on the lookout for new usable details. Disguises allow him access to conversations he wouldn't otherwise have heard and to situations he would not have ordinarily seen. This leads to a deeper understanding of the mission. People unknown to him will bring him the details that take him to the next step. He knows that he will have to sacrifice his time and energy and ask difficult questions of people he may not yet know.

Ethan Hawke wholeheartedly accepts the mission every time. For him, there is only one way to go, and it is forward. I need you to do the same. Look toward your ultimate goal of better health. Continue to remind yourself of your key motivators. Your relationships, your family, your dreams, and your desires are waiting.

Sometimes Ethan Hawke is beat up along the way. You may feel beat up at times too. But the triumphs you experience will far outnumber and outweigh the disappointments. Small steps made in the direction of your goal lead to greater understanding. Taking action based on that new understanding leads to small successes. Small successes over time and with commitment lead to revelations about your healing. Revelations confirm that you are on the right path. Staying committed to the process and accepting new information as it is revealed leads to triumphs.

When you first start on the mission, it seems like you have no path and no direction. It may appear that you have no way of finding the answers. You may feel alone. You may have had disappointments. I know. I have been in your position. Many people have had similar frustrations even though their specific health challenges are different than yours. You and I will take the steps together, one by one, to start Mission You.

The first task is to modify the internal questions you ask yourself. Changing the questions you ask will change the answers you receive. If you choose to accept this mission, the path of healing will begin to take shape in front of you. The choice is yours. The mission is there. It is waiting for you to accept it.

Ask Better Questions

Have you ever thought, or wondered aloud, "What is *wrong* with me?"

"What is wrong with me?" is a nonproductive question. You may as well be asking, "Why is it cloudy today?"

Reporting on the current conditions has some limited value, whether it is your symptoms or the lack of sunshine. Regarding your symptoms is good; it gives you a place to start. But we need to be more targeted in our questions. New, properly phrased questions will illuminate your path and move you away from the dead-end questions. The one and only way to solve the mystery and complete Mission You is by moving forward step by step, with intelligent purpose.

When you ask better questions, your brain gives you better answers. I know it sounds simplistic, but many of us habitually ask defeating questions. Very often our questions are subconscious and may be rooted deep in childhood. You may have prejudices that are not your own but belong to your parents. (As in, "Why don't you go to a *real* doctor?") You may have an unconscious spontaneous tendency to overdramatize. (It could be that as a child the only way for you to receive a little extra needed attention was to pretend to be sick or overemphasize symptoms to appear sicker than you were.) You may have an unconscious spontaneous tendency to wonder what pill you should take. (Such as, "Are you *taking* something for that?" Or, "Do you have a pain pill? I have a headache.") You may panic yourself into thinking that your issue is quite clearly an emergency and you need an immediate medical appointment or urgent care. (For instance, you have had a cough for three weeks and on Sunday at four p.m. you suddenly believe that it is worse and deserves a chest x-ray at the local ER.)

Our old habits may have been useful in the past. But now, you are on a mission to change. In order to have a breakthrough, you need to be willing to break something.[51] Said another way, to allow yourself a new direction on a new path, your habits need to evolve. Being stuck is just that, stuck. A whole new life waits for you. Be bold. Strap on your flak jacket. We're going in.

---

51 Credit Tim Ferriss, American entrepreneur, author and podcaster.

The Looming Lupus Diagnosis

Claire was hoping, as we all do, that she would go to the medical doctor, they would look at her, look at her blood test results, and say, "Ahhhh. I know what all of this is. Take this prescription twice a day for three weeks and you'll be better." You go home and resume your life. Done.

You know the story didn't happen like that. As is true for most of you who are facing a health challenge, this doesn't happen a lot of the time. Usually it takes three appointments, two blood tests, waiting for results, one CAT scan, two more appointments, an ultrasound, and a referral to another specialist.

Unfortunately for Claire it became worse. After two blood tests, a normal brain MRI, and the referral to the specialist, she was told, "You might have lupus. Go arrange your life."

The day I met her she was with her two young boys, ages three and four, who were testing out their Spider-Man skills on the chair with wheels, my exam table, and my computer mouse. Claire's eyes were so bleary she could barely open them even though we turned off the lights. Her feeble attempts at telling her boys, "Stay still, don't play with that, come here next to me," resulted in zero response from them.

Lucky for her she was in my office. A friend told her, "Go see Dr. Nancy, just go." This was after she had done her online research on what to expect of her life with lupus. She was horrified. Over the last six months, she'd had constant dizziness, extreme fatigue, eye pain, and headaches. According to the lupus research she had done online, that would only become worse with time. Claire's internal questions were dragging her deeper into depression. "It must be my fault. I must not be cut out to be a mother. It's too much; they said so. It's too stressful for me. Why did I do this to myself? My husband must regret marrying me..."

Her husband, Derek, did have his own frustrations. Claire said, "He's worried about me, for sure, and wonders how he'll have time to care for me and the boys. They aren't doing homework yet but one day they will. Who's going to help them do their homework if I'm in bed all the time? How do we get through the day? And Derek has his business to think about too. He said that he might have to go back to his corporate job if I don't get better.

Then there's the Disney trip. The boys are just old enough to love it. But I can't even think about planning it. The thought exhausts me."

She had been to the M.D., she had a prescription which means she should be better, right? She began to ask other questions: What if the symptoms weren't real? What if the symptoms were all in her head? She should just snap out of it. Because to look at her, she was a beautiful young woman. How could there be anything wrong? Or at least anything wrong to this severity.

Day after day the symptoms remained. All the wishing did not make it go away. Claire blamed herself. Quite obviously, she believed, there was something she should've done, or shouldn't have done, that would have prevented this diagnosis and kept her from being a burden, rather than the mother and wife she had planned to be.

Here's the thing… Here's the very important thing about Claire: she listened to her friend. The sad truth is that if she would have asked her medical doctor if chiropractic would help with her lupus diagnosis, I would bet the answer would have been a solid "No." And keeping the answer simple, he might have added, "And don't see a chiropractor." But Claire didn't ask her medical doctor. She trusted a friend.

I was her last-ditch effort to find some path of healing. The last resort. She had almost no faith that her investment of time and money would result in anything with chiropractic. But I did. I knew. My evaluation told me that there were opportunities for healing and improvement. I knew Claire could heal even when she didn't. In nearly all my encounters with new patients, as well as my encounter with Claire that first day, I visualize them a month in the future after we have completed a treatment plan. I can visualize them feeling freer, with significantly less pain and discomfort, able to live life as they have wanted. I don't share this visualization with most because they have spiraled downward so far, they no longer believe that they can heal.

Claire improved with her chiropractic care dramatically within the first few weeks. Her final blood test results, which took two months to obtain, showed inconclusive results. She no longer believes that she has lupus. Her symptoms resolved one hundred percent within four weeks of our meeting. She and her husband and the two boys have a trip planned. They leave for Disney tomorrow.

Your Diagnosis is a Label

Claire's story shows how disabling a diagnosis can be. Simply put, it is a label attached by The System. When you've been told you "have" something, the curiosity stops. It disengages your desire to ask the better questions. When you're labeled, it's like saying "game over!" Mission complete. Discontinue searches. Discontinue thinking. Discontinue any path of healing. There's only one way to go, and that's down. The downward spiral of debilitation, of explaining your disorder to people so they understand your limitations. Detailing to the kids why you have to sleep in and can't take them to the park, or why Disney is just a thing that other families do. Shamefully telling them that, once again, you had to leave the school play or football game early because you had one of your "cluster migraines," or that you can't help with the senior banquet as you had planned because your BPPV (benign paroxysmal positional vertigo) is too severe for you to drive. That's what a diagnosis does. It classifies you as a completed System project. And if you are complete, then there is no mystery to solve, and no mission.

It's not that your diagnosis is wrong. It may be completely accurate. Or, as in Claire's case, completely off the mark. Mentally it stops you from the exploration for true healing. It closes off options that could restore you.

Think of Mission You as an alternate way of thinking: you reject The System label. You choose to believe that you are whole and healthy. Some challenges need to be addressed, absolutely. But you know there is a better way. And you are right. Let the search begin. Let's learn how to find those better options. Right now.

Powerful Question #1: What If I Could Heal?

The System wants you to believe that you are broken. The System wants you to think that only the magic in a pill or potion or going under the scalpel could possibly reduce the pain or discord that runs your everyday life. That it and it alone holds the answers. The kicker? The System has either chosen to ignore or forgets that your body is a self-healing miracle.

Of all the things you will learn from me, the following one modification is the most important: **What if I Could Heal?** This question is to open your eyes, and help your brain be receptive to the multiple answers that exist. **What if I Could Heal?** means that you're not willing to take a proton pump inhibitor for heartburn the rest your life. You won't endure a mouthguard for TMJ syndrome indefinitely. You're not going to succumb to the thought of neck surgery, you're not going to be satisfied that physical therapy helped reduce your pain by half, to just be resigned to your problem. You're not going to endure hot flashes and sleepless nights, urinating just a little when you laugh, and decreased intimacy with your husband just because everybody else says it's normal. You're not going to accept that the pain in your foot, a diagnosed condition of *plantar fasciitis,* will only be placated by cortisone shots. You're not going to agree when a medical doctor says nobody can help you... Merely because *they* can't help you... And, while you're at it, why don't you see a psychiatrist.

What if I Could Heal? reveals that you are in awe of the human body, that you know the body can make huge healing strides if given the chance. If given the building blocks it needs and if interferences in body function are cleared, your body has the best chance to change and heal. We have been so bamboozled, even brainwashed, via all those ridiculous commercials that drugs are the only choices. Or, that our choices for managing symptoms are drug A versus drug B versus drug C. We think that's the choice in healthcare. Nothing could be further from the truth. A world of opportunity for health and healing is available, and we have that information literally at our fingertips.

Did you ever shop for a new car? You never owned a Honda before, but you've heard good things about it. After a test drive you tell the salesperson you'll need to think about it, and what is it that you see on the road at stop signs, at red lights, going in the opposite direction on the turnpike? It's that same Honda you test drove. It is everywhere. You hadn't noticed before how popular it was. In actuality it was there the whole time. But now your brain has been cued to look for it. You weren't purposefully looking for Hondas. It's just the way your brain works. So, asking the question **What if I Could Heal?** allows your brain to look for the clues and be open to the unexpected discoveries. You may not understand the relevance of the information you're receiving, or the purpose of the people that suddenly appear in your life. Merely asking **What if I Could Heal?** allows the people, the agents of change, the ancient manuscripts, and the covert intelligence to pass through that open doorway. And you are ready and waiting.

Better questions give you better answers. **What if I Could Heal?** presents new possibilities for you. Ask this question and it could be life changing for you. Answers are within reach. Resources of people, books, and concepts are right outside your back door. They wait for you to be ready to discover them. My promise for you is that you will be on your first steps toward healing. This is it. This is the very first step. *If you get nothing else from this book, simply asking this important question will alter your trajectory.* Embrace this question as your personal crusade, and I will have achieved my life's purpose of helping to unravel Mission You.

Powerful Question #2: **Why?**

The second question to ask is **Why?** because it opens up the ability to learn. It isn't a "Why me" question. That, my friends, takes you nowhere. It's a "What is going on with my body?" and "What series of events have led me here?"

For me, when I was dealing with the gremlin in my gut, a necessary tidbit of information was sent to me by my mother. She was in the process of moving from the home of my childhood, and she bequeathed me a composition book with my name on the front. My mother kept meticulous notes of the medical interventions of my older brother, my sisters, and me. She recorded every doctor's visit, every medication, notated with the date and the outcome. This ancient manuscript created by my mother held a secret. The new intel contained a clue that led me on the path to healing my gut.

In 1972, I was in the first and second grade. I vividly recall the matching outfits my mom made for her and me, particularly the green pants suit. Mine had given me the nickname Jolly-Green-Giant because of the plaid green top and pull-on pants. That, and I was nearly the tallest girl in my class. I also remember being in Dr. Dubin's office. He was our family doctor, and we would walk the four blocks to his office in Franklin Square, New York, which was on the lower level of his home. The midcentury white tile floors had a reflective shine and there was the clear, sharp scent of rubbing alcohol. By reading the composition book with the black and white cover on which my name was written in pencil, I learned that when I was seven years old, I was on antibiotics seven times.

In the early 1970s it wasn't known that the overuse of antibiotics would lead to lifelong problems and drug resistant bacteria. We didn't know that even one course of antibiotics leads to an imbalance in the natural flora, our own good bacteria in the gut. Antibiotics were in its heyday. It was the miracle drug. The 1970s were a time when moms brought the kids to the doctor for every sniffle and cough.

This did not dramatically affect me until I was 35 years old. And it seemed sudden and came without warning. But those symptoms, I learned from this memoir, did not come out of nowhere as it had seemed those many years later.

If I had not been asking **Why?**, the ancient manuscript would've held no secrets. But because I was asking, my mind was open to new information. In the quest for **Why?** nothing is ignored. Small details revealed in the unfolding scenes of any mystery often become pertinent later on. Because you play the leading role in Mission You, you are not at the whim of a family member, a health professional, or a well-meaning neighbor. You are on a mission, and it is the most important job you have. Your life as you know it, or knew it, needs you. Your dreams and desires want to become reality.

Once you start to ask **Why?**, your intention for everyday life changes. No matter if you're speaking to a neurosurgeon, a gynecologist, a health food store operator, or an energy medicine practitioner, you are always allowed to ask that question. Asking a neurosurgeon about your neck pain might lead them to say it is there because of a previous car accident that affected your neck. Asking the gynecologist about that same neck pain, albeit likely a holistic gynecologist, may prompt them to say that you may be estrogen dominant, which might cause joint pain. The nutritionist might say that you have an inflammatory response and to try taking a turmeric supplement. The energy medicine practitioner might say that because the neck houses the fifth chakra and you've not been able to speak your mind, there is blocked energy there. You may accept, or reject, for now, any of these reasons. But each deserves investigation.

The Effects of Stress

Every day you encounter opportunities to mess up your body. We abuse ourselves with an overabundance of environmental stresses and still stomp through our daily rituals regardless of the effects.

There are at least three types of stress in our daily lives: physical, emotional and chemical. (A fourth is electromagnetic, and I'm sure there's others.) Physically we traumatize ourselves constantly. Our bodies tolerate poor sitting postures at desks and in cars. Getting into car accidents, micro- and macro-repetitive trauma at our jobs, sport injuries, falls, and caring for children, whether you are a twenty-eight-year-old mom, or a sixty-four-year-old grandma, add to it.

Our world is inundated with psychological turmoil. Emotionally we worry and beat ourselves up over issues we cannot control. None of these stresses put us in any real physical danger, for the most part, but our body perceives it and reacts to it as such. The detrimental chemical cascade that occurs in our body when we are exposed to prolonged negative events doesn't depend on there actually being a saber tooth tiger waiting to eat us, we merely need to *believe* that a metaphorical saber tooth tiger lurks. The effect is the same. Our body can't tell the difference.

We chemically stress ourselves with foods laden with additives, medication, alcohol, cosmetics and beauty products, and cleaning solutions. Then there's the things we can't control: agricultural pesticides and herbicides, mold spores, chlorine and contaminants in our water, and a potpourri of industrial and petroleum fumes. Despite all of this, our body keeps coming through for us. We pick ourselves up, dust ourselves off, never taking time to recoup from the damages. Because we don't listen to the symptoms or we use medications to dull them, our bodies stop communicating the need to pause, regroup, and repair. Other organs or body parts take over for the failing or malfunctioning pieces. We then compensate for those compensations. It is a spiral that, unless we choose a healing path, continues down and down. When you take a discerning look at the symptoms you experience and recount the events that led to your illness, you help in your quest for healing. Looking at current circumstances could reveal what underlying forces are at play.

There is the distinct possibility that your body is doing something right. It may be a response to an activity or change that you have recently made. What was that? Like me, you may be dealing with residuals from a childhood medical intervention. Or, it may be a repercussion of tolerating an issue that started long ago. Have you been ignoring symptoms? Or have you been chalking it up to the usual excuses: you're the migraine type, you always get sick this time of year, your dad had IBS so you will too, your doctor told you there were no other options besides medication, all your friends get hot flashes too, the list goes on. Is your body doing something in response to a threat, such as a germ: bacterial or viral or parasite? Does your home or work environment contain toxic molds or heavy metals? Is there a long-standing weakness for which you have been compensating? Is your body doing something wrong? Some respond by saying that our body is never wrong, that protection of the individual's life is paramount. But with protection, a choice is made by your body to choose the priority of preservation of life, and new weaknesses are created. Did you have an injury as a child, recently, or long ago? It could have required a dramatic emergency room visit, or not even close. What was the mechanism? Do you recall the specifics?

There are lots of questions to ponder, I know. This book is not designed to magically impart all the tools that I have after a doctorate degree and twenty-five years in a busy practice treating 20,000 different people. But take heart. Asking yourself this second question, **Why?**, will allow new illuminations to occur. Once you start asking, this question gives you permission to uncover clues. You allow yourself to start digging through your personal history. You look for interdependencies between organs, accepting your body for the vitalistic structure that it is. Every tissue and organ is dependent upon the other. No effect of excess stress is left without leaving a telltale footprint.

When you accept Mission You, you don't get all the details, at first. Asking the question **Why?** puts you in discovery mode where no tidbit of information is without value. You just might not be aware of its importance when the scenes first play out. You are like *Mission Impossible*'s Ethan Hawke. Everything is important. No doors are closed. All can be opened. Every clue has relevance. Store the information away. You are on a quest. You are on Mission You.

Powerful Question #3: Where Are My Resources?

Powerful question number three, **Where are my Resources?**, requires phys-ical action. Because you started this journey by asking the first two powerful questions, you are now ready for the third. You have shifted your mindset, see your health conquest from a new perspective and are ready to assem-ble your healthcare arsenal of people, gather reliable resources, and make measurable improvements in how you feel. While the enemy has been an influence in every move you've made your whole life, allies are all around you waiting to help with your issues and to help you break free of the con-fines of The System. But they are in stealth mode like you.

Jason Bourne of the movie *Bourne Identity* awakens from his injury-in-duced coma onboard an Italian fishing boat. He has no recollection of where he is, who he is, or what events led to his being there. The one clue is found on a small laser device implanted in his hip. It leads him to a safety deposit box that contains money, weapons, passports. He chooses a name from the pile of passports he finds there. Realizing that he is in danger, he recruits someone for support. This is his first ally. With the items found in the safety deposit box, and the street smarts of his ally, he navigates his way to other people who give him additional information. Each encounter, whether it be the fight at the Paris apartment or the shoot-out in the countryside, leads to the next step of discovery.

You are in the same position. You are waking up to The System's influ-ence. The System is all around you attempting to affect your thinking and your actions. The billboards on the way to work along the busy boulevard for the women's health center. The ad in the friendly community magazine for the neurology group. The three-page spread about the new Alzheimer's drug in your favorite print magazine. The banner and side panel ads of your online search engine for medications you don't need with the very fine print at the bottom that, if you were to read it, warns you of the dangers of taking this route. The television show with the young handsome hero in the smock of an MD with angelic qualities of unending compassion and apparent mystical insight. The gossip magazine at the grocery checkout whose cover boasts the "Ultimate Weight-Loss Secret" alongside the can't-miss recipe for Super Fudge Belgian Waffle Cake.

Awareness of these subtle, nearly imperceptible pressures of The System to conform and the insidious dangers that lurk within is the first step to new discoveries. Like Jason Bourne, you are awaking from an apparent coma and will begin to unravel your mystery by reaching out to your first ally. The first person who is of help to you may simply show you a commonsense approach, or direct you to an author, or a book, or expert. Slowly you will gain confidence and momentum as you uncover additional elements of healing. Asking, **Where are my Resources?** tells your subconscious that you know you are able to heal. That confirms that you trust yourself more than the entities of The System. Remember that if the normal or conventional had gotten you to your destination, you would not be looking for alternative routes. There is a solution and you are on the path to discover it. Usable details will start to flow in. You are savvy enough now to research typical treatments and the meanings of diagnoses. You have already begun to ask yourself the first two powerful questions (**What If I Could Heal?**, and **Why?**) and that puts your brain on the lookout for usable details. Soon, people now unknown to you will reveal themselves as allies in Mission You.

No Matter What, You Can Do This

Right now, as you are sitting here reading this book about the monumental changes you can make, I want you to speak a word or two of gratitude. You might be grateful for a realization that you've been messed up for a long time, or that you've made some missteps along the way. That's okay. Or, perhaps it's that you've recently taken some positive steps toward healing. Maybe you have a supportive spouse or friend that deserves recognition. Whatever it is, take a moment and shout, whisper, or mutter aloud your gratefulness. When you are done with that, thank yourself for being the bold creature who picked up this book. If someone recommended *Stealth Health* to you, thank them. Saying this out loud sends a message to your subconscious of your unbridled commitment to Mission You.

I know all this can be daunting. As you travel on your individual path, you might feel like you are alone. You are not. As you explore, allies and helpers will make themselves known. You can take this journey with their help. I'm going to show you how.

You may think that you don't have the smarts for this. I am telling you that you do. We all do. And here's the funny part. A thorough understanding of anatomy and physiology isn't necessary. The greatest scientists of today admit that we have only scratched the surface of understanding the mysteries of the universe, and the intricacies of the human body. A healing method doesn't require its mechanism to be known for it to work. Many of the greatest healing techniques produce wonderment at their power from the practitioners themselves.

It takes faith, I know. But you have, until recently, put your faith in The System, the people and places that didn't pay off. And now, I'm asking you to put your faith in the one place where the person won't let you down - in yourself.

I've seen hundreds, if not thousands, of people regain their health and fulfillment in life by taking ownership and using these steps. I, personally, have taken these steps. Come along with me for Mission You. Big changes are coming. Whenever you doubt yourself, remember this: The System taught you to say and spell *acetaminophen*. You can learn anything.

Mission You: Take Action

- **What if I Could Heal?** Start with this most powerful question. Meditate on it. Pray on it. Use it as your waking thought of the day and your final thought when you fall asleep. Open up to the possibilities of what it would take to heal. It is the greatest step you can take. If you do nothing else in this book, then do this.

- **Why?** Contemplate your history of illnesses, your genetic background. Ask questions about your past to those that know you. Ponder the possibility that choices made by you or made by others on your behalf have brought you to this place. Knowing from where you came and retracing your steps can give you the fuel to make corrections. Looking back to see the faults of the past will help you to not make those same mistakes again.

- **Where are my Resources?** Start compiling a list of your known resources. These can be people you know, or people that you would like to meet. Family, friends, friends of friends, healthcare professionals, healthy people, people trying to make healthy changes, even the weird guy at work that eats only broccoli.

- Because most of us have poor memories (it's not just you), download two things from my website, *www.DrNancyTrimboli.com*. The first is *Mission You Journal pages*. Print and carry one with you to jot ideas, people's names, and online sources to check. The second is *My Healthcare Arsenal* spreadsheet. As you become aware of people and professionals supportive of your ability to heal, add them to your list. When you are facing a health challenge and not feeling well, check back to this record. It's crazy how, in our darkest moments, the pain, disease, or fear can make us forget what will help most. Use this as your memory.

- Have you found a great resource? Is it a professional sympathetic to your frustration with trying to heal within the confines of The System? Do they have a healthy skepticism for The System? Is it a website or an online professional that has helped someone you know? Is it a book that was recommended from a reputable source? Share that information on our *Trimboli Insiders Group* on Facebook. Not a member yet? You'll find a clue to entry at the end of Chapter 3.

Chapter 3

YOUR NEW RESOURCES

People, Books, Online Searches, and
Unexpected Discoveries

From Seven Medications to Zero

"WHY AM I taking this?" Mark wondered aloud. And, without consulting anyone, even his wife, he started the deliberate process to eliminate *seven* medications.

Mark's story is a common one. His father and uncle both had heart attacks at a young age, which meant that he had a family history. Being an achiever type, he had excelled as a top advertising executive, a baseball coach, a dad of four boys, and a big game hunter. He had his first heart attack at age 49. When I got a chance to speak with him, he told me that the approach was to take seven medications.

"They told me that I had a heart attack, so I must take all this medication. They called it the *standard of care*," Mark said. "My concern was that I didn't want to be dependent on those drugs for the rest of my life."

He continued, "Those meds, they really changed my brain health. Being in a state of irritability with my wife, family and coworkers, and the mental fogginess that went along with it, made every day difficult."

I remember him saying that he contemplated the worst, meaning suicide without saying "suicide," working out details of the when, the where, and the how. He knew that the change in personality he experienced was completely attributable to the drugs.

"I'm still a bit foggy," he said, "but what it did more than anything was curb my confidence in public. I need to speak in front of groups all the time for my job. While on those meds I would ask myself in the middle of a presentation, A*m I saying this right? Where do I go with this?* My command of the room was shot."

"On the inside I would be fearful and trembly. Afterward I'd beat myself up for not being as sharp as I'd like and thinking my performance was poor. Then at home I'd be in a sour mood and my kids didn't want to be around me."

This is the medical algorithm at work. The algorithm directs patient care. Treat the diagnosis, not the individual. But here is where the adherence to convention stopped. Mark started to ask **What if I Could Heal?** He wasn't willing to be a lemming and follow the common protocol that put him on seven medications. The System was right there in his face, in his Sunday-through-Saturday pill organizer that he had grown to hate. He asked better questions: What is this medication doing to me? Why do I feel so bad? Why am I on this medication? He started to track his blood pressure. He had never had high blood pressure. As Mark took his readings twice a day, and started to reduce the blood pressure meds, his diastolic and systolic numbers didn't vary. His decision? Stop taking it. He got positive reinforcement from a new medical doctor, who did not adhere to the seven medication rule for the first heart attack. Then Mark allowed himself to be bolder when he asked the question: **What if I Could Heal?** He researched the other medications. He researched heart health and nutrition. With his new intel, he made life changes, adding supplements, and became deliberate about his food choices. One by one, being careful to monitor his vital signs as he went, he removed the next six medications. He became a Stealth Health operative.

Mark's experience would be a fun story if you didn't have any other background information. It becomes a tragic story when you know the torment that the medications were causing him. At *AskAPatient.com*, a common cholesterol-lowering statin drug is rated 1.8 out of a top rating of 5 with 887 patients giving feedback.[52] Immediate side effects include anxiety, memory loss, nightmares, severe leg pain, shoulder pain and neck pain, difficulty walking due to severe foot and leg pain, dizziness, and fatigue. Mark was troubled by most of these. Yet his first medical doctor did not monitor those side effects. Switching to his second cardiologist, who had a different approach, put Mark on the mission to research for himself. He watched YouTube videos, he bought books and read them. Today he is off all his medications. Mark feels like he has regained his life, his family, his livelihood, and his sanity.

"My boys no longer run out of the room when I get home. That's a blessing."

Immediately after his heart attack, Mark had no idea that he would change cardiologists. He had no idea the devastating effects the medications would have on him. The books that contained the ideas that changed his life were formerly unknown to him, even though he had a genetic predisposition for a cardiac event. Mark hadn't been interested in becoming a healthcare expert in any fashion. But life handed him a challenge. Accepting the challenge has turned it into Mission You. Mark's mission is not over, although the mystery may be solved for now. He may face challenges in the future and will need to be vigilant of his condition throughout the rest of his life. But to his credit, his first steps put the power of his own health back in his hands, removed the dangerous side effects of medication, and secured expert resources to continue to learn and grow. Mark asked better questions, got better answers, and was unraveling the mystery of himself.

Cardiac health and the prospect of having a cardiovascular event, like a stroke or heart attack, evokes fear in many Americans, as it should. It is the leading cause of death worldwide. The number of deaths due to cardio-vascular events is expected to increase by 50% by the year 2030, in spite of the projected medical treatment costs in the U.S. to increase to over $700 billion dollars by that time. If the medical treatment worked, why would the number of cases and the cost be increasing? If we want to reduce cardiovascular events and deaths, perhaps the answer is not in distributing more medical care.

---

52 www.AskaPatient.com. Accessed October 19, 2019. https://www.askapatient.com/viewrating.asp?drug=19766&name=ZOCOR.

At first, Mark felt defeated and had no hope. The medications accentuated this feeling by increasing his anxiety and depression. Luckily some part of him wanted to win, to find a better way. He began to ask the powerful question: **What if I Could Heal?** A shift in mindset, in perspective occurred. Mark believed that he could heal. He was open to new information when a trusted friend referred him to a medical doctor with a holistic approach. Changing cardiologists was a key for him to regain his confidence. Just as you will discover for yourself, this healthcare professional became a resource for him. The new mission was to remove the drugs from his life and, most importantly, improve his cardiac health.

Nothing was spoon-fed to Mark. He did the work, the reading and the research. There is power in knowledge, especially about yourself. As Mark continues to learn and gain clarity, his lifestyle choices will be deliberate. Future treatment choices will be made not out of fear, but with confidence. Mark became an expert on *Mark*.

As we continue through this chapter, you will discover that, like Mark, you have a wealth of health discoveries waiting for you. Your new health resources will stem from multiple places.

Face-to-face interactions with local professionals who have dedicated their lives to helping people will give you great insights. Friends and family may have an arsenal of indispensable healthcare professionals that, before now, they didn't see the need to share with you. People in your life will step forward with great leads to follow. All you need to do is start asking the right questions. The shift in mindset takes only a moment.

Get into the habit of buying and reading books that pertain to your health issues. Clear off a shelf in your home. Keep books, like *Stealth Health*, close at hand. You will be referring to this book and others for reminders as you heal.

While we are in a new world of information gathering, The System has a stronghold on how readily you can access or research anything that is contrary to it. Your internet searches need to have a specific landing page for a trusted source. Rather than a general search by topic, target specific landing pages of people, books, films, podcasts, and videos. Once there, use other links to guide you along.

The ability to be open to unexpected discoveries can be life transforming. Avenues of life-changing ideas will come at you from the most unlikely places. I'll clue you in to the ways to be observant.

There is a movement afoot. The System may be strong and have infiltrated our lives. But coming to your rescue are authors, filmmakers, researchers, journalists, holistic healthcare providers, and whistleblowers willing to put themselves at risk to defy The System. Their messages are gaining traction and their voices are growing louder. All you need to do is learn to look and listen.

Your Healthcare Arsenal: People

"Shoot, I can't eat this," I said. "It's got vegetables in it."

I was sitting across from Susie at a restaurant booth. I had known her for years, and we'd been through more than a few emotional roller coasters together. She is a massage therapist, a really good one, and a bit of a hippie. If you want to know the location of a sweat lodge where vision seekers meet the second Saturday during the summer months, she's your gal. Who would have thought there was a shaman teaching in the distant Northwest Indiana suburbs? Susie introduced me. We went to classes with the shaman to experience rebirthing through hyperventilation and finding your totem animal guide. It was pretty cool stuff for somewhere between the Sears Tower and cornfields.

Seeing as how I said, "I can't eat vegetables" without thinking, I was a little startled by Susie's response.

"What does *that* mean? What's wrong?"

It is a rule for me not to discuss physical ailments with anyone, particularly digestive issues, over lunch. But I soldiered on. I had only discovered recently about the vegetable thing, so I laid out the details of my story leaving out the most embarrassing parts. I felt like I could trust her with my story because she is a healer who knows things that I don't know. She knows a shaman, for one. For a fact she discusses issues with her own clients during their massage time so there's probably not too much that she hasn't heard.

I was right in telling Susie my story. She made a suggestion. I didn't ask her for it, but she is a helper-type person and freely shares her knowledge.

I do have to admit that when she told me her idea, I was not open to it. The type of healthcare practitioner she recommended was a type that I had heard bad things about. Not from anyone that actually used this practitioner's service. Which is not fair. I had a prejudice against a whole healing art because of one thing said by one person. That could have limited my healing. But instead of holding onto that false belief, I took her advice. That moment was a turning point for me. It was the first thread of unraveling the mystery of me. Other components would need to be addressed, don't get me wrong. But if I had held onto that false belief, and rejected her idea because of it, my mystery would remain unsolved.

Susie is a person who is a resource for me. People in *your* life are resources as well. Up until this point you may not have needed the information. As a massage therapist, and a hippie, Susie has a unique perspective. She understands the innate healing ability of the body, and she has seen miraculous changes in people with massage therapy. She is open to alternative methods. Notice that Susie did not recommend a massage technique for me. It was a colon therapist which helped my issues. You would think that as a chiropractor working in that alternative healthcare field, I would be aware of *all* the alternative techniques. Apparently not. If I was not aware of it, there is no way that you would have heard about it either. Unless you have a Susie in your life.

It is likely there are people in your life very similar to Susie. They may or may not be in a profession that is in a healthcare field. They may or may not appear as a hippie. You may notice them at family parties eating different foods than everybody else. You may know that they have been down the road of an illness and recovered. They may have a child who is special-needs. These people may be resources for you to help find the turning point in Mission You.

Your job is to find data that's been hidden from you, so don't discount the oddballs either. "Oddball" means that a person swims upstream against the current. The reason your family giggles about your Wacky Aunt Edna behind her back is because she is different. This may be exactly the kind of resource you're looking for. Someone who operates on a different level. Someone who has seen things that the rest of the family has not seen. She has broken ties with the norms of your tribe. She has made discoveries and followed her own path, adhered to her own set of rules. Aunt Edna may be a great resource for you. Or, she just might be bats.

Tap into all the resources you can muster. Your spouse or your best friend may have a chiropractor. You may know someone from the gym who works at a health food store. Your sister's best friend may be a doula. Ask around. Great sources of information are right outside your back door. Don't be surprised if, when first asked, your neighbor's daughter can't remember the name of the reiki master she saw. Encourage her to let you know when that name pops into her head. Follow up with her. Mission You is your priority because regaining the life you want is primary. No stone is left unturned. No witness is left not interviewed. This is your path of discovery and all informants are called to testify.

Should you enlist a local healthcare provider to be part of your arsenal, give them information about what that means. On my website, *www. DrNancyTrimboli.com*, download the workbook page *Stealth Health Provider Guide*. Encourage them to reach out to us. They'll get the scoop on how to help you and how to become part of the Stealth Health movement. It's you, our patients and clients, that will topple The System. Providers that are now in the shadows need to band together. Your involvement will implement that. Thanks in advance.

Navigating Uncommon Sources: Books and Online Searches

This is it. Having accepted Mission You, you ask better questions. Imagine yourself like Sherlock Holmes, the sleuth, who ponders and speculates. Attack this mission with fervor. Working deeply undercover, you will meet strangers in the dark. (Likely on your computer late at night. Your face aglow with the artificial white light coming from the monitor.) Because you are interrogating these strangers (or their websites) for information, there are specific questions to ask. Gathering intel is the job at hand. As you are reading, you may come across phrases or words that are confusing. Jot on your *Stealth Health Secret Intel* journal pages those concepts or words that you can't quite grasp. As you discover new information, you will gain greater insights into these. Learn about you. Learn about your normal function and also about your dysfunction. Become a Stealth Health operative.

The Ancient Language

Latin is used by medical professions so that they can communicate across languages, much like botanists and biologists do. However, the language divide can also separate you from understanding your body and your issues. This is a way The System uses to trick you into thinking that your health and healing are outside of your control and your understanding. The System wants you to believe that only the magicians in white coats or matching scrub tops and pants have the intellect to translate the ancient language. With my help, you can and will be able to learn enough to discern the meaning of Latin terms.

The most important thing right now is Mission You. Focus on what you can learn rather than what you do not know. Allow things to unfold before your eyes. You will have a greater understanding of you than any doctor can ever have. I promise.

Latin translations of your health issues are called a *diagnosis*. Having a diagnosis of *gastritis,* or *spondylosis,* or *plantar fasciitis* does not give you any clues to answering your three new powerful questions: **What if I Could Heal? Why? Where are my Resources?** Latin translations of our symptoms to form a diagnosis is designed to help a medical doctor with their algorithm. A diagnosis leads to a prescription for a medication much of the time. If you are labeled with a diagnosis, you may consider it a piece of the puzzle, not the solution. A diagnosis is far from a solution. It is a label; a label written in an ancient foreign language.

Learning the ancient language is not without value. For one, we need to be able to converse with members of The System and speak their language. When you meet with members of conventional medicine, it can be helpful to cite a diagnosis with which you've been labeled. Scheduling appointments is easier when the receptionist has a diagnosis. It doesn't help members inside The System to know all the details you hope to uncover, especially those that make your appointments. The level of severity of your problem or diagnosis may not grant you extra sympathy, but it will make communication easier.

The second reason is to know how The System would treat this diagnosis. This is important to know. Research this. The System may have a perfectly safe and effective option. Educate yourself to have greater understanding. Learning about the conventional medical path will tell you if you want to investigate that route. Conventional medicine may only have limited tools at its disposal, meaning medication or surgery. Be able to accept or reject such treatment.

If you are not willing to accept medication for your problem at this juncture, don't make an appointment with a medical professional, unless it is a functional medicine or holistic practitioner. Search another line of clues. Showing up in a conventional medical doctor's office and announcing that you don't want medication will only cause everyone to feel uncomfortable. Support staff of medical doctors will be disarmed by your request and won't know what to do with you.

Get used to seeing the alien Latin, Greek, and German word roots associated with the organ that is needing your attention. In addition, there are big, long names of biochemicals racing through your body. You don't need to memorize these but try to gain understanding of the building blocks of chemical reactions and processes. Write these things down on your *Stealth Health Secret Intel* pages for reference later. Look for diagrams if that helps. Look for a crash course that breaks down the complex concepts into easy to understand pieces. Don't be afraid to search for the kindergarten version of things. A profound interconnectedness of organs, tissues and cells exists. Body parts that seem distant from your issues may have an intimate connection after all.

When attempting to become an expert on your problems, you may need a friend to translate complexities. *Mission Impossible*'s Ethan Hawk didn't need to know how to hack into computers. He had a buddy back in the van talking into his earbud. After he sashayed into the cocktail party and tiptoed away to the hostess's home office, he could confidently do his work with the instructions being whispered into his ear.

Cracking the code

Begin where you are today. You may have no background in human biology, but, darn it, The System taught you to spell and pronounce *acetaminophen*. You can learn anything. Because you don't know what you don't know, get some basics first. Start with general knowledge about the organ or body part where you have problems.

Let's use as our example: acid indigestion. Start with some basic facts. In one of my favorite resources, *Encyclopedia of Natural Medicine* by Michael Murray and Joseph Pizzorno, Dr. Murray explains normal body functions, abnormal functions, what the typical conventional medical treatment entails, and holistic options and why those may be a better choice.

This Encyclopedia is over one thousand pages, and, if you are a nerd like me, you read it cover to cover. But we aren't reading it for fun, we are reading to discover. If you're not sure where to start, open the book to the index. The index is in the back of the book. It lists all the topics or important words in the book in alphabetical order. Look for symptoms or start with a relevant chapter. Since our topic is acid indigestion, I first read the chapter *Digestion and Elimination*.

No matter what you are researching, be sure to not only read, but study. Take notes. Keep a journal of your discoveries. While reading the digestion chapter, I stumble upon a fantastic concept. Dr. Murray writes, "many nutrition-oriented physicians believe that it is not too much acid but rather a lack of acid that is the problem." Wow. That is a novel concept. The lack of enough acid in my stomach makes me feel acid indigestion. I read ahead to the next section titled, *Hypochlorhydria*. That's a big word. I use my online search engine and find the definition of hypochlorhydria. It tells me it's a syndrome of not enough stomach acid. *Hypo-* means less than normal, *chlor-* is the root for hydrochloric acid (HCl, the chief digestion chemical in the stomach), and *hydria-* is a liquid environment.

Okay, now for the second powerful question: **Why?** As I look up the definition of hypochlorhydria using my search engine, I scroll past the sites where The System has a tight hold. They have domain names similar to these fictitious ones: health-arrow, medi-doc-on-the-web, mustard-clinic, ducknoisewatch. I would tell you the exact domain names to avoid, but like I said, we are keeping our heads down, staying undercover. You, and I, are in stealth mode for a reason. Going out of my way to mention these by name may draw unneeded attention to ourselves, and we have other priorities right now. The priority is solving Mission You.

Going back to the search, I see an article with a simple title, *What is Hypochlorhydria?*[53] This particular article is on the first page of search results. Like I said, all the links on this first page may be controlled by The System,[54] but I click on it anyway. I read the article, and it makes sense. It contains the symptoms of hypochlorhydria, the reason someone would have it, and the good things to do to fix it. In most well-written articles about health topics, footnotes indicate the research or other authorities from which the author obtained information. By scrolling down I see the sources. In this instance these are hyperlinks. I click on one called *Gastric Balance: Heartburn Not Always Caused by Excess Acid.*[55] The title pretty much says it all. In the article it states that hydrochloric acid (HCl) produced by the stomach decreases because of age. (In a moment we will discuss Dr. Murray's perspective on this.) It's an interesting article packed full of facts. Routinely, until about the 1920s, it states, excess stomach acid was fully treatable with supplemental HCl which was recommended by medical doctors. However, for their own reasons, doctors stopped recommending HCl. The author quotes Dr. Johnathan Wright, a Harvard graduate medical doctor and advocate for patient freedom of choice in healthcare. Dr. Wright says, "Encouraged by the ... drug industry, medical students are not taught that hypochlorhydria (inadequate stomach acid production) is treatable ... with unpatentable, natural replacement therapies. Instead, their education concentrates on hyperchlorhydria (excess stomach acid production) and its treatment with patentable acid blocker drugs and highly profitable over-the-counter antacids."[56]

I had to read that last quote of Dr. Wright's five times before I under-

---

53 "What is Hypochlorhydria?" *Healthline.com,* Accessed July 25, 2019. https://www.healthline.com/health/hypochlorhydria.

54 Gray, Bryce, "Round-up Lawsuits Shed Light on Monsanto's Internal and Controversial PR Strategies," *St. Louis Post-Dispatch*, September 2, 2019. Accessed September 7, 2019. https://www.stltoday.com/business/local/roundup-lawsuits-shed-light-on-monsanto-s-internal-and-controversial/article_c58f814f-f3c6-5aef-badb-c9b59b113e42.html.

55 English, James, "Gastric Balance: Heartburn Not Always Caused by Excess Acid," *Nutrition Review*. November 25, 2018. Accessed July 25, 2019. https://nutritionreview.org/2018/11/gastric-balance-heartburn-caused-excess-acid.

56 Tahoma Clinic, Medical Staff. Accessed July 25, 2019. http://tahomaclinic.com/medical-staff-2/dr-jonathan-v-wright.

stood the meaning. I'll rephrase it in case I lost you somewhere. At some point about one hundred years ago, medical students were no longer taught that too little acid caused heartburn and indigestion. Schools also stopped teaching about the cheap fix of supplemental HCl. Instead, the lesson that too much acid was to blame provided a reason to prescribe a profit-generating chemical. Their education was modified to render a diagnosis that would prompt the use of a drug, whether that was the proper treatment or not.

Fascinating, right? In researching, I found a way to help myself, and I've also found a way that The System wedged itself in between people and an effective, inexpensive, safe option that would help them. Because HCl couldn't be patented (it's a lab-produced combination of naturally occurring elements), it is therefore not profitable. The result? Medical doctors were no longer taught of its effectiveness. They were only taught about the diagnosis of *excess* stomach acid so that they could recommend a profitable prescription drug.

I would stop there, but there is one more point to be made. Proton-pump inhibitors, a class of drugs commonly prescribed for acid indigestion, were shown in a 2018 research study to increase the risk of pneumonia in adults over sixty.[57] The drug doubles the rate after six months of use and triples the rate of pneumonia after twenty-four months. This is significant. For the last hundred years, The System has hindered and sickened people by infiltrating itself into the education of doctors. The drugs cause increased illness. Fascinating and appalling at the same time.

As I continue, I search for the top books this year on the topic of digestion. Increasingly, a leader in a new concept, or a safer healing method, writes a book and has resources for your specific problem. Others, who conquered their own health challenges, are sharing their experience and paving the way for you. For me, that search led to some great books with topics that had never occurred to me. I might investigate further and buy a book on leaky gut syndrome, how gut health affects hormone balance, or healing my gut with a G.A.P.S. diet.

Finally, I go back to the Encyclopedia of Natural Medicine to continue reading about hypochlorhydria. Dr. Murray gives a detailed explanation on

---

57 Zirk-Sadowski, J et al. "Protein-Pump Inhibitors and Long Term Risk of Community-Acquired Pneumonia in Older Adults." *Journal of American Geriatrics Society*, 66, no.7 (2018): 1332-1338, Accessed October 19, 2019. https://doi.org/10.1111/jgs.15385.

how to take HCl. So I'll go to the local health food store, purchase HCl for less than fifteen dollars, and start to heal myself.

Even with all this information on hypochlorhydria and a strategy to help, it's only the first step on my journey. I'll start taking the HCl according to Dr. Murray's instructions, but there may be further **Why?** answers for me. Once I receive the books I ordered and read those, I'll discover the next directives to explore on my mission.

This story centers around acid indigestion. The same steps can be followed for infertility, high blood pressure, kidney stones, gout, migraines, mood swings, insomnia, menopause symptoms … any health mystery that Mission You needs to solve.

Booby Traps to Avoid

You aren't going to find good information easily. You will have to search for it. Network, cable, and local television will not have it. Nor will commercials, banner ads or web-based news headlines, or major news outlets. Those are all controlled by The System.

As a Stealth Health operative, you will be collecting this newly discovered intelligence. Record your findings in your workbook. Copy web addresses. Make paper copies of particularly sensitive information. The System may remove it.

With Mark and his cardiac issues, his path of discovery was initiated by his cardiologist. First were Dr. Sinatra's book, *The Sinatra Solution*, the documentary *Statin Nation* featuring Malcom Kendrick, and the book *Statin Nation* by Justin Smith. Taking the time to watch the film and read the books led Mark to greater understandings of his cardiac health.

In both cases, the origination of the search began with an expert. In my case of acid indigestion, the expert was author and naturopath, Dr. Michael Murray. With the cardiac health search, it was Mark's holistic family doctor. If you try to start the search by jumping into the quagmire of internet keywords, you may become lost. The first page of searches is where The System leaves traps for you; snares to lure you back. Most people stop at the first page. Go to the second, third, or even the fourth page of search results to find true gems.

As you surf around the internet, searching, looking, reading, watching videos, you'll find that many people want to sell you their vitamin line. This is a diversion tactic. Don't fall for it. Supplements may become a big part of your life, but now is the time for gathering information, not jumping into bed with the first pretty girl you see, no matter how many 007 movies opened with that scene. Use the information that supplement websites may be offering about products and the reason the product was developed. Passionate people with a message to share put time and effort into business launches with the creation of their website, content, and products, then developing an audience. Their products may be excellent but resist the urge to dive in at first glance.

When you are internet searching, try this for a brief comedy intermission. Search anything holistic or natural-health based with the word "scam." It's entertaining to see the dramatic drivel that pops up. For every one advocate for holistic care, it seems there are three active website creators pushing out contradictory trash every day. The bigger the alternative concept, the greater the target for its detractors. Come to expect it. I even go so far as to think that the more negative articles I can find, the more beneficial the topic. Try it just to get yourself used to it. It's The System at work. Try searching: earthing mat scam, or pediatric chiropractic lawsuit, or epigenetics hoax. Keep in mind that statements are misrepresented as facts and plain truths are twisted. I've included footnotes for positive articles.[58,59,60] You'll have to do the scam search yourself, just for the fun of it.

---

58 Oschman, James, Gaetan Chevalier, and Richard Brown, "The effects of grounding (earthing) on inflammation, the immune response, wound healing, and prevention and treatment of chronic inflammatory and autoimmune diseases," *Journal of Inflammation Research 8* (2015): 83-96. Accessed July 25, 2019. doi: 10.2147/JIR.S69656.

59 Shaw, Gina, "Safety and Effectiveness of Pediatric Chiropractic," *ACA News*, April 19, 2016. Accessed September 27, 2019. https://www.acatoday.org/News-Publications/ACA-News-Archive/ArtMID/5721/ArticleID/165/Safety-and-Effectiveness-of-Pediatric-Chiropractic.

60 Lipton, Bruce, "Epigenetics 101," *YouTube*. Video File. June 26, 2016. Accessed July 25, 2019. https://www.youtube.com/watch?v=G4T0LzU_rv0.

Unexpected Discoveries

The woman to my left in row fourteen of the flight from Atlanta to Chicago points to my water bottle as I chug the last ten ounces. I see her lips move but I can't hear what she's saying. Actually, I think she's just mouthing the words until I realize that my earpods are still playing the wave noises I fell asleep with.

I yank the pod out of my left ear and smile, giving her that squinty-eyed look with a head tilt that we all know means, "Excuse me, what did you say?"

She asks, "May I ask you about your neck pillow?"

I say, "Oh sure," and we chat about that. I dig in my purse and pull out a business card to write down the title of one of my YouTube videos. "I've done a plane travel video where I mention this specific pillow," I tell her.

Her eyes widen as she looks at the card.

"You're a chiropractor. (*Pause.*) A *chiropractor.*" She looks off into the distance as she says this, her mouth slightly slack, literally a look of awe.

She finds the words to speak. "I was just thinking … And, I don't know if a chiropractor can help me … But only a moment ago, I was thinking, when I get to Chicago, I need to find one. But still, I don't know if it would help. And … it turns out that I'm sitting next to one!"

This, my friends, is an unexpected discovery. She was thinking it. And there I am. Crazy, right?

I inquire, "Tell me what's happening?"

She explains that perhaps from wearing high-heeled shoes for many years in the corporate world, or from who knows what, she has a deep pain between her second and third toes of her right foot. When she puts pressure on it, like with walking, it's intense.

As she talks, I look down at her feet and see that indeed she is wearing flip flops. Not cheapy dollar ones that no one should wear, and not the cutesy ones all us girls wish we could wear all year long. They are very *functional*, in a very practical color of brown with a touch of tan. The thong part of the shoe indents the white socks that I presume are needed more due to the coldness of the plane and not some homage to her apparent Asian ancestry. Considering her beauty, youth, and the meticulous eye makeup, I'm sure it is disconcerting to reduce herself to such footwear.

Then, as if on cue, I see it. The look of unsettledness that I see increasingly often, because what appears like a simple issue has treatments that are completely undesirable. These conflicting thoughts wear on the common sense of your psyche.

Then she says it. "My options are a cortisone shot that may work temporarily at best, or a surgery to cut the nerve but a new pain could start at the stump, or to wear the only shoes that don't give me pain." Admitting that the elder-wear were the best option seemed to have completely exhausted her. This was illustrated by the heavy sigh and the slight frown.

I explain that the pain she is feeling is commonly diagnosed by conventional medicine (including podiatry), as a neuroma.

"Yes! That's what they said!" She reacts like I had just read her mind. (I was on a roll with that apparently.)

I went on to explain that a chiropractor could determine if the L5 nerve of the lower back was causing some or all of the problem with her foot.

"They'll be able to know that?" she asks.

"Oh, yes, definitely. All chiropractors are trained to do that." I continue, "Also, there's a chance that it could be misalignments of the foot creating a problem."

"Really?" she says, "They can correct that?"

"Yup. Absolutely."

"Ya know," she says, and I could see the mental wheels turning. "My boss is always bragging about her chiropractor and how it's like magic; the things he does for her. The thought nagging me is that there's got to be a better way. But, what is it? What is the better way? This may be it. I'm going to reach out to him."

I reflect on the way she posed her powerful question, **What if I Could Heal?**

"Excellent. It sounds like you are on your way to healing," I said.

And she responds. "Yup. Absolutely."

As you are lumbering along, a gem may drop from the sky like a big fat raindrop. Or you may be flying through the sky and a pearl of wisdom might emerge from the mouth of the chiropractor sitting next to you in row fourteen. Discoveries like this will seemingly appear out of the ethers, but you'll be ready for them. Because you have been asking the three powerful questions, your brain is alert and on the lookout: **What if I Could Heal? Why? Where are my Resources?** Good questions lead to insightful answers that change your life. This gem could be the secret to the success of Mission You.

That new idea, at first glance, may stagger you with its simplicity. You may think, how could it be this simple? Why didn't someone explain that to me? Or, if is something that you've had success with previously, how could I have forgotten this? It is possible that this intel was there before, lurking in the shadows. Just like my row mate, she had heard good things about chiropractic. It was in her mind to look for a better way. And there I was. A reminder.

The powerful questions put you in an open state of mind. For me, my earliest powerful questions were for my patients. Early in practice, well before the "raisin" medication incident, a representative for Meridian Valley Lab introduced me to testing for delayed food reactions which could create joint pain, asthma flare-ups, sinus issues, even ear infections and mood swings. (To be clear, delayed reactions are an immune response of IgG antibodies as compared to IgE antibodies which are immediate and severe reactions. It's two different immune pathways.) This was new information for me, but I was always searching health-generating ideas for the good of my patients. Using myself as a guinea pig was my usual mode, so I did the test. It came back with some surprises. And, as you may have already guessed, it turned out to be an unexpected discovery in my own healing.

Here's the pertinent back story. Most of us have tangled webs of health issues, and I am no exception. I had my first sinus infection when I was sixteen, although I didn't know what it was. I just knew that my face hurt. My second sinus infection was at about age twenty-eight and was rapidly followed by the third, the fourth, and so on. The only way to stop it was antibiotics, which troubled me. I was actively searching for answers, but those seemed elusive. I struggled at times with fevers that came in waves, and feeling fatigued.

My results on the delayed food allergy test showed a sensitivity to the nightshade plants. This family of plants includes tomatoes, bell and hot peppers, eggplant, and potatoes. All of my favorites. So, what the heck, let's follow Paul's directions. Paul was my rep who introduced me to the test. He has since passed away, but I am forever grateful that he strived to help people, and for his motivational words to me: "This could solve many of your patient's chronic pain problems."

With my test results in hand, the next step was to eliminate all foods containing nightshade plants for two weeks. Then, eat a meal containing one of them.

So, okay, I thought, *Let's give it a whirl.* After my two-week drought I ate tomatoes on my salad. Within an hour I had a sinus headache. None the previous two weeks, then *BAM.* Of course, I didn't believe it. How could I have a sinus headache from a tomato? I've been eating tomatoes my whole life! Blast, it can't be. Let me wait a couple of days and try it again. *Bam.* Same thing, except worse. Like, lay down in a dark room worse.

As I test each of the foods in the nightshade family, I find that peppers cause the sinus infection to return. It's not just a headache. One small taste of a pepper made me sick for five weeks. Five weeks full of pain, lethargy, gunk, and mucous. I had found my **Why?** Eating a bell pepper will create a sinus infection.

Of course, I don't just accept this. I attempt to undo the allergy. Over the years I've tried various reiterations of NAET (Nambudripad's Allergy Elimination Technique) with only a temporary ability to eat peppers. But still, I must ask: **Why?** It's not until years later, after the "raisin" medication event and my eventual gut rebuild that it all makes sense.

Let me weave that together for you. The excess antibiotics I used as a child caused a candida overgrowth in my gut. Candida, or yeast, is a one-cell organism that has tentacle-like projections. Once it takes up residence in your intestinal lining, it creates large gaping holes to allow undigested food particles to be available for the yeast to eat. The problem is that if a food particle gets into the bloodstream before the yeast can eat it, the immune system sees it as a foreign invader. Your white blood cells attack it and remember it for future encounters. For me, there must have been a piece of green pepper that was the innocent but targeted culprit. As soon as the white blood cells sense that same invader, meaning, when I ate a bell pepper, a battle was waged. Immune response spiked inflammation of my sinuses, and, when severe, became an infection. As crazy as it sounds, the sinus infection that I had at sixteen was the first sign that I would have intestinal problems as an adult. This is just one illustration about distant body parts having an intimate connection.

Luckily all of this is behind me and I am grateful for all the various healing discoveries I've made. But if you have a chili cook-off in my honor, I probably won't attend. Even the aroma of cooked peppers in the air will give me a headache. If I'm at your house for your son's graduation party, and I don't eat at the taco bar, please don't be offended.

Along the way to heal my leaky gut, I was researching apple cider vinegar when I stumbled upon the G.A.P.S. diet book by Dr. Natasha Campbell-McBride on Mercola.com. I ordered the book, read it cover to cover, and dove in. Through the G.A.P.S. diet of food elimination, reintroduction of foods, bone broth, and fermented foods, I rebuilt my intestinal wall. It was the secret to my healing that took nine months to completely sort out. Even initially, though, I knew it was helping.

You will have your own unexpected discoveries. The receptionist at the cardiologist office may offhandedly mention a magnesium supplement for your heart palpitations, although your doctor never did. A magazine cover at the local health food store may connect joint pain and statin drugs. Your mom may mention that Wacky Uncle Wally used to make ginned raisins for his arthritis. A conversation you overhear at a restaurant may enlighten you on the possible dangers of root canal procedures. The class-parents of your son's third grade room may be discussing the supplement that rid their sons of warts. Your hairstylist might be showing another stylist an exercise to help with her arm numbness, that you try, and it helps with your carpal tunnel symptoms.[61] A word spoken by a stranger, stumbling upon a concept while online, or a book with unique ideas may be the start of something beautiful. Follow the radiance of the gem long enough to see if it leads to greater understanding. Be vigilant. Sometimes the lesson you need to hear is one that's been told before. A news story headline may jostle a neuron in your brain that is on the lookout for clues. A recollection from an old friend about problems you fixed earlier in life may rekindle a memory of a previous path that worked. It could be true you have taken a supplement

---

61 Trimboli, Nancy "Median Nerve Stretch." *YouTube*. Video File. May 12, 2018. https://www.youtube.com/watch?v=D8aqK3-obHk.

or seen a health provider that helped you for this same issue in the past. Pursue that same course of care again.

The System loves the idea of one diagnosis, one treatment.[62] It's simple. But you know this level of dysfunction did not happen in a day. Even if you have found what you think is your complete answer, it may not be. As with me, you may find you pursue a path that was unknown at first. Often, an undercurrent of health challenges was brewing that were nearly imperceptible. Over time, your poor body struggled to maintain some semblance of normal for you. You keep pressing on every day with the job, with the peanut butter sandwiches for the kids' lunches, and with the mortgage payments, all with a smile. Other organs may have jumped in to compensate for you. Some organs became collateral damage. Clues may uncover the fact that additional healing must be done. Just because Jason Bourne found his passport with his name on it, that didn't stop him from unraveling the entire mystery. Enemies were on his tail, the mystery was waiting to be solved, with side stories to make it interesting. Just like you. Never stop searching for clues.

Gaining Momentum

At the beginning, you may be unsure of what information, people, or resources to trust. That's understandable. Health problems are rampant, and for the enterprising, a source of never-ending income opportunities. In Chapter 6, I will share strategies on how to discern the resources to follow from those to be wary. For now, I just want you to start gathering intel. Reach out to those people in your circle of friends, family, and peers who have resolved their own health issues. Ask questions of the staff of your medical provider, as often they listen to the stories of patient successes more raptly than the doctors themselves. Attempt to recollect the healthcare providers that you or your family members have seen who you may consider as being outside of The System.

If you are lucky enough to have a long-standing relationship with a

---

62 Occam's Razor states that the simplest explanation is most likely. In contrast, Hickam's Dictum states, "A man can have as many diseases as he damn well pleases."

healthcare provider who may be outside of conventional medicine, make a mention to them about your new quest. Often they are able to offer an immediate trinket of information that starts your journey. I find that my own patients are not fully aware of all the skills I possess or the problems that can be helped by chiropractic. I am thrilled when patients approach me by first saying, "This is probably outside of your field but, do you know anything about _____?" And most times, I do. I consider it my duty to be the catalyst for your healing. On the rare occasion that one of my patients does not respond to our care, I gladly refer them to another healthcare provider that I believe can help them. Those of us that work stealthily outside The System know each other, or at least *know of* each other. From my office, we not only refer to conventional medical doctors, but also to functional medicine doctors, acupuncturists, homeopaths, energy medicine practitioners, colon therapists, wellness physical therapists, nutritionists, Ayurveda doctors, chakra balancers, and reiki masters. We are also familiar with resources in the form of books, podcasts, online experts, and websites. Seek out the healthcare providers in your circle. Give them a chance to make a difference for you in regaining your health and your life.

With the internet we have a world of opportunity of health and healing literally at our fingertips. There are thousands of people wanting to help with the health challenges you face, and they use the internet to get a message through. For them, it is a huge undertaking to develop and focus their message, create a brand, and build an audience. Most of those people who have undertaken the challenge to build their business online have their own history of problems that propelled them into the healthcare arena. It is always better to start with a good source on the internet and use their hyperlinks to seek additional content. Or, find valid information via an author who supports true healing and alternative disciplines. If you do an online search for specific authors, you can access information that they share. I would caution you against books that have a purely medical perspective or that do not discuss holistic or non-conventional medicine approaches. Some authors specifically warn you to *not* investigate alternative approaches. Unfortunately, these books aim to corral you back into The System.

Do heed the following warnings, however. Avoid conversation threads in chat rooms. I have rarely seen valid advice in amateur chat rooms. User comments on expert websites, which are posted mostly by non-credentialed persons, can distract you from the mission, so be wary. As always, a personal referral by a friend is best, whether to a new health provider in your community, or to an online expert.

There are fantastic books on health and healing and I'll be sharing my favorites with you on the Resources page at *www.DrNancyTrimboli.com.* Continue to check back as you progress on your healing journey as new books are added to our list all the time. There is a surge rising as people, like you, realize that The System needs to topple.

Your Work Remains a Secret

Throughout Mission You, you will mostly keep your discoveries and your work a secret. This mission is yours. Although you travel alone, you will enlist the help of others along the way. They may be a true ally, a resource that you can go back to repeatedly, or it may be someone on their own mission, parallel to yours. Once you find that ally or resource, keep them close.

You will need to steal snippets of time to follow up on leads and research clues. You may need to stop whatever you are doing to jot down the domain name of a podcast you are listening to. Or you gather intel under cover of night while the house sleeps. That crucial phone call from a local holistic practitioner will have to be answered as the 2:30 bell rings while waiting on the pickup line at the middle school. The covert operation has begun. Put on your aviator sunglasses, get out your shoe phone, and put that hidden camera in your lapel. We are now in Stealth Health: Mission You mode.

Mission You: Take Action

- If you haven't already done so, download *My Healthcare Arsenal* spreadsheet from www.DrNancyTrimboli.com. Add to your list of your resources compiled in Chapter 2: acquaintances, doctors, health providers, massage therapists, teachers, pastors, friends, family, your wacky Aunt Edna, chiropractors, reiki practitioners, energy healers, the yoga teacher at the YMCA. As you become aware of people and professionals supportive of your ability to heal, add them to the list. If you are someone that's not crazy about recording things like this, don't worry about it. The three powerful questions will carry you through.

- Fill in details on the *My Healthcare Arsenal* Excel spreadsheet: the date, their name, special talents or training, and what intel they shared with you. Ask about their resources: people, internet sources, books that made a difference for them, everyday habits that they swear by. Write those down.

- Teach yourself about your problem. Purchase a good book to use as a reference. See www.DrNancyTrimboli.com for my favorites. Download the *Mission You Journal* pages from my website to document your discoveries, or, if it feels right, specific things of which you are grateful for each day.

- Keep a record of informative websites and books that you have referenced. These also become part of *My Healthcare Arsenal*. Having OneNote, Evernote, or some other online content capturing app will save time. Be sure to review your findings often.

- Are you ready for a reward? We reserve access to our *Trimboli Insiders Group* on Facebook for those of you that have invested your hard-earned money in our books or courses and shown a commitment to take back your power and unravel the mystery of you. By buying this book, you have done just that. And you made it through Chapter 3! Be proud of yourself. You are learning and ready for change. Connect with me personally and with our community. Share your new favorite resources. Others are working on their own missions in secret on a parallel path alongside you. Sharing your favorite sources can help someone unraveling *their* mission.

Go to www.DrNancyTrimboli.com, look for the hidden hyperlink in the book title, Stealth Health. This will give you access to our *Trimboli Insiders Group* on Facebook. As long as Facebook groups, my website, and hyperlinks exist, it will work.

Chapter 4

USE MEDICAL TESTING TO YOUR ADVANTAGE

WHEN YOU STRUGGLE with an issue, it's easy to say "yes" to any prospect of help. But now you have accepted Mission You and are armed. You've been asking better questions to discover better answers. You have your newly discovered resources. With some critical information your next steps will become evident. Medical testing and technology can help.

"Eliminate him." As Jason Bourne in *Bourne Identity* recovers from his amnesiac coma, he is unraveling the mystery of his identity. He gathers intelligence that reveals he is a soldier in the plot to assassinate someone he has never met. The enemy, which is his own government and employer, will stop at nothing, even to the degree of expending the lives of other agents, to eliminate him. Jason Bourne realizes, through clues left behind and conversations with allies, that he does not support the agenda of his enemy and boss, or the methods they use. Once having recognized it, his mission is to free himself from their clutches.

In your case, the enemy is The System. You are the expendable foot soldier that is led to believe you are incapable of comprehending the complexities of your own body. The System has an agenda of its own. The underlying motivation may be unclear but for it to be the strongest, it requires you to act on faith. You are kept in the dark, believing yourself to be dependent upon it. Commandeering your own health choices that are outside of its influence creates chinks in its armor. Only if we stay within the confines of The System, subdued and agreeable, does it survive.

Conventional medicine is part of The System. The Latin terms, unreadable handwriting of a prescription, and the lack of understandable terms move you away from knowledge. It removes you from a position of power and makes you an underling. Your opinions have little bearing, and you are tricked into thinking you haven't the intellect to understand. Only the wizard in the white coat can understand. You are a peon and a serf. That's what The System wants you to believe. But you are on a mission. Taking back your knowledge of health and healing gives you the power in your quest to solve Mission You.

In Chapter 2 you learned new, better, and powerful questions: **What if I Could Heal? Why? Where are my Resources?** With those, you summon specific answers about your path of healing. This gives you momentum. You are gathering facts, and you have created an arsenal of resources. Knowing that you were previously a pawn in The System gives you new perspective. You have exposed hidden truths. This new awareness puts control in your hands. You have ammunition. Your perspective now is that doctors, nurses, technicians, and all the support staff *work for you*.

Walking into a medical doctor's office with Mission You in mind puts you in the stance of data mining. You may humbly realize that you need to gather information from those with greater understanding than you. Or, on the other hand, your ultimate destination of true healing may not include what your medical practitioner has to offer. In this case, you may want to consider the option to use blood tests, blood pressure screenings, MRIs, ultrasound tests, bone density tests, x-rays, and other medical tests to give you information. You may use those as a starting point, a baseline, or as a way to check progress as you travel along your health path.

Finding alternative ways to heal yourself without medical or pharmaceutical intervention is detrimental to The System. You have seen others around you whose lives are dictated by medical appointments, to the degree where their whole schedule is filled. Sometimes they relinquish their ability to choose and just follow doctor's orders without understanding the ramifications, side effects, or outcomes of recommended treatment. Their lives are changed forever because of a surgery gone wrong, or a medication perceived to be the only choice. You don't want that for your future.

On the other side of the spectrum, you see other people making better choices and asking better questions. They are able to free themselves from the burden of health issues. Like them, you feel that medications should only be used on occasion, not as a lifestyle choice. That's what you want for yourself. It doesn't matter if your ultimate goal is to ride your bike when you are eighty, or still attend that ten-day yearly fishing trip with the guys in Saskatchewan. You want the freedom and independence to live your life as you wish, not be tied down with doctor's appointments or a timer to remind you to take your pills. It's not that you are looking for anything grandiose. You live life as you dictate, doing the things you love to do. Losing your ability to make true health choices is linked to losing your inalienable rights as a person.

How to Approach Medical Tests Like a Boss

The way you arrive at your medical doctor's office is important. Put on your flak jacket of knowingness. You know you have an issue. Medical testing *may* reveal some clues on your healing path. It may not. You are not there for a white slip of paper, although you may accept it graciously, knowing that you might never use the prescription. And, you are not there for useless tests. If a test will bring clarity that helps you on the next step to solve Mission You, follow the prescribed protocol. Using expertise of someone who can discern test findings and show you a next step would be helpful. You are not looking to be labeled with a dead-end diagnosis.

Foremost in your thinking are your three powerful questions: **What if I Could Heal? Why? Where are my Resources?** Prior to arriving at your appointment with the medical professional, you have outfitted yourself with information that you procured from other sources. You may have discovered it on your quest while working stealthily undercover, covertly from the internet, from reading and understanding a book or a chapter on the subject, or from another health professional. If you should undertake medical testing, it is for one reason. It is to derive information about **Why?** this issue is happening with you, and postulate answers to **What if I Could Heal?**

Gathering Intel – The Four Medical Testing Questions

When faced with the recommendations to do medical testing, there are four questions you should be asking. Go to my website for a free downloadable page of questions to bring with you to appointments. Jot down the answers as soon as you are able.

1. "If the recommended testing results in normal findings, then what is next?" (Options might be further testing, the same treatment as if abnormal results were obtained, no treatment but merely a "wait and see," or referral to another conventional medical provider.)

2. "If the results of this test come out abnormal, what does that mean?" (Possible answers are the same as above. Options might be further testing, the same treatment as if the results were normal, no treatment but merely a "wait and see," or referral to another conventional medical provider.) When testing is recommended, it usually means that the outcome will either confirm or rule out a diagnosis. *Rule out* is a term that means a particular diagnosis is being eliminated based on the test. For example: Doing a swab of your throat will either confirm or *rule out* a strep throat infection. Other questions to ask would be: "What are we looking for? What are we ruling out?"

   Note: If the diagnosis, underlying cause, or options of treatment *do not change* based on the results of the test, *do not have the test performed.* Testing should only be done to discern a path toward treatment or healing. If it does not, it has ceased to be a benefit to you. It is a benefit to The System.

3. "In what way will the results of this medical test direct treatment options for me? What benefits or adverse side effects can be expected from those treatment options?"

   a. If drug treatment is recommended, "How long will I be on those drugs? Short term? Or indefinitely?"

   b. If surgery or another type of intervention is recommended, "What is the recovery time? Can I expect to need another surgery or intervention of this type again in the future? How will my life be changed if I have this done? Would you recommend that I get a second opinion?"

4. "How invasive is this test? Are there any dangers to this test? Does a different, less invasive test give me the same or better information?"

In the medical system, the primary treatment options are medications. If this is the only reason to have the test done, and you know that you will decline drug therapy, it is worthless to have the testing done. If you unknowingly accept the testing and subsequent treatment without having a firm idea of the path conventional medicine will offer, you have just submitted to the bondage of The System. On the other hand, being aware there are other avenues for healing you could seek in the alternative realm puts you in control.

The System wants you to be in the cycle of diagnosis that leads to medication, and side effect symptoms or syndromes that lead to a new diagnosis and associated medication. It is a rare medical professional that wants to remove drugs from your list, and an extremely rare individual that wants to eliminate the entire list of medications. If you find a medical professional that insists on removing drugs from your life, and will assist you in doing so, keep this person close. They are a Stealth Health ally and have elevated themselves to a resource. Write their name on your list.

If you find that you have good rapport with your conventional medical professional, you may ask, "Is there an opportunity to use holistic care, a nutritional regiment, and are you aware of any drug-free alternatives?" Medical doctors unfortunately see the world as it has been taught to them. They are forced into The System similarly to you. Don't fault them for this. It has been ingrained into their procedures, policies, and behavior for decades.

Being part of the corporate medical conglomerates subjects many medical professionals to the stresses of audits both governmental and corporate, quotas to reach or risk having their income infringed, and increased patient volume to make up for fees slashed by in-network insurance plans. Medical doctors have agreements with other local providers to refer patients back and forth to help each other with quotas. An orthopedist may have a relationship with a rheumatologist since patients may present to both with similar complaints of joint pain. It gives them an opportunity to create income through multiple office visits and to order medical testing.

If you have an opportunity to ask, "Is there are any conservative or holistic avenues that I could or should explore first?," be warned. Once you mention a holistic care paradigm, alarms may start going off in the head of the healthcare professional. They may offer phrases such as, "I think there's some good in some alternative methods." Or, "My wife is a health nut too." Or, "One of my other patients sees a chiropractor, and it seems to benefit them." Or, it could be, "Stop looking things up online." Or, "Whatever you do, don't see a chiropractor." It can vary.

There are exceptions to the rules of conventional medical care, and great healers know that there are many methods to healing, not just the tools in their own toolbox. Alternatives within conventional medical care are emerging, with functional medicine being one of them. The amount of experience with alternatives are still up to the individual doctor. Not all people, and not all doctors, work the same. If a medical doctor does tell you to avoid alternative treatment, ask them if they have had personal experience with it. Not hearsay or stories, but firsthand experience. Only by being a patient of an alternative healthcare provider can you really understand what it can do. Even if they have experience, and especially if they have none, their opinion is a personal opinion, not a professional opinion. Unless they have earned a chiropractic degree, they cannot say if you are, or are not, a candidate for chiropractic care. Just like a chiropractor cannot look at your teeth and tell you if you need braces.

Singular Focus on Mission You is Paramount

Your singular focus on Mission You is to not succumb to the rhetoric of The System. The System needs you to follow its rules, don't ask too many questions, and, for Pete's sake, don't look for additional information on your own. The System doesn't work if you are overtly on a mission. This would turn people off, make them suspicious of you. The conventional medical office staff may label you as a troublemaker. Your Stealth Health strategy is to look like you belong, like you are a lemming following all the other lemmings. You may accept a white slip of paper for a drug only if you see this conventional medical office visit is a dead-end, and you wish to exit the office without drawing attention to yourself. At times we may need to act like we comply with recommendations just to avoid extra scrutiny. That's why it's a Stealth Health mission. Not everybody understands our mission. It's not our place to explain it. Take the white slip of paper, smile, and retreat into friendly territory.

No matter how open-minded your medical professional, there is an ingrained prejudice to holistic care methods. This is not new. It goes back to the time of Hippocrates and the ancient Greeks. Two schools of thought related to healing and the human body emerged at that time: mechanism and vitalism.[63,64,65] Mechanism espoused the perspective that the human body could be divided up into parts and studied. Today's conventional medicine sees health and healing as mechanistic, as though the human body were a machine whose parts work independently from each other. This is the reason for specialties within medicine, for example: cardiology (heart), immunology (immune system), orthopedics (joints and bones), and dermatology (skin). Mechanists also believe that the diagnosis directs the treatment, not the individual with the diagnosis. Therefore all people with a diagnosis of heartburn are treated with the same medication, everyone with tension headaches is given the same recommendations, everyone with spinal arthritis is treated the same, and on and on.

Vitalists, on the other hand, believe that the body has an inherent life force and an intelligence that goes beyond our human understanding, and that the totality of our body is greater than the sum of the individual parts. Every person is an individual, with unique needs for their healing. Focus is on assisting the body so it can do what is intended and heal itself. Homeopathic remedies use small amounts of a toxic substance your body

---

63   Coulter, Harris, *Divided Legacy: A History of the Schism in Medical Thought, Vol IV* (Berkley: North Atlantic Books: 1994), 666-692.

64   Bradley, Rachelle, "Philosophy of Naturopathic Medicine," in *Textbook of Natural Medicine*, ed. Joseph Pizzorno (Amsterdam: Elsevier, 2012) 61-68.

65   Coulter, Harris, "Empiricism vs. Rationalism in Medicine" *The Journal of Orthomolecular Medicine* 9, no.3 (1994)

is fighting to increase the fight from your body. A chiropractor may adjust your back or neck or even your foot to help the lower back pain that keeps you from standing up straight. An acupuncturist looks at your tongue no matter what illness with which you present. The vitalist approach does not require a diagnosis because it addresses the imbalances that interfere with the normal recuperative power. Your body does the rest.

These two schools of thought are still active today. You may use both schools of thought in your path of healing. You may see a chiropractor because getting your upper back adjusted helps with your asthma symptoms and also have a medical doctor prescribe an inhaler to use routinely or as needed. You don't need to choose sides. Some doctors within the mechanist or vitalist worlds may tell you that you need to choose a side, but that is not necessary. Many aspects of modern conventional medicine are useful and safe. These can work alongside most holistic remedies. Unless there is a logical explanation given, don't let anyone tell you otherwise. This is Mission You, and you know best.

The Dreaded Ear Infection

The fear on Luke's face belied his six-foot, five-inch height. His usual Nordic blond calm demeanor became one of a frightened five-year-old. He was worried. The pain he had felt in his ear for the last two days, so bad that it was keeping him awake at night, was reminiscent of the ear infection pain he had as a child. He came to me with this issue.

Luke had recently played a backyard volleyball game, after which his shoulder bothered him. It was that shoulder on which he had surgery during his college baseball days. It had never been the same after surgery. Luke had been working for me as my assistant for six months and knew that the chiropractic adjustment could work miracles. He and I discussed the volleyball game and the ear pain. Perhaps that was the **Why?** Perhaps the two were connected. I found a muscle on the side of his neck that, when in spasm as it was, could trigger a phantom pain in the ear.[66] The spasm

---

66   Davies, Clair, *The Trigger Point Therapy Workbook: Your Self-Treatment Guide for Pain Relief.* (Oakland: New Harbinger Publications, Inc.: 2004), pp. 51-55.

could have resulted from too many volleyball serves using the already weakened shoulder.

I did an adjustment of the shoulder and our massage therapist worked the muscle. Sam also used the cold laser therapy on his ear to decrease the pain he was feeling. We repeated that for two days. He was no better. The ear pain was still keeping him up at night and he was worried. Repeated antibiotics used for ear infections on Sam as a child affected him now as an adult. He told me he very much wanted to avoid antibiotics.

As he said this to me I could see the underlying question **What if I Could Heal?** written on his face. After the bodywork course of action had failed, we needed more information. Luke made an appointment with a nurse practitioner at the local urgent care. She confirmed it was, in fact, an ear infection.

Luke took the white slip of paper for the antibiotic prescription from her but did not fill it. On our next workday together, he came back to his resource, me. With this new information of the confirmed ear infection, I recommended colloidal silver for its antiseptic action. He took it orally and also put two drops in his ear a few times a day. Two days later, the Luke I knew was back. Ear pain gone, sleeping through the night, and no longer worried.

In this case, supplemental information was needed to take the correct path of healing. Luke started at an easy entry point, the chiropractic adjustment and massage. Consulting with me was easy to do because we worked together. His first course of action, meaning the chiropractic adjustment and muscle work, had benefit but did not solve the ear pain. By seeking a conventional medical professional, he gathered needed intel that confirmed the presence of an ear infection. The intel helped him choose another path.

Luke did not bother the nurse practitioner with the information that he had tried the bodywork (chiropractic adjustment and massage) with no help. He merely told her the symptoms that he was feeling and let her do her job. He also did not share that he would not fill the prescription for antibiotics. Sharing that would be of no benefit to him or to the practitioner. He was in Stealth Health mode. He knew the reason he was at the conventional medical office. He was there for information. The information allowed him to reach out to his resourceful person (me) for help in a new course of action.

There is a world of opportunity for health and healing. Using medical professionals for their expertise and the testing is our right. If you arrive armed with information and options, you can make completely informed decisions. Don't feel disappointment if their only option for you is medication. Remember that's their job, to name a disease and treat the disease using drugs and surgery. They are ingrained in The System. You are breaking free. Get the intel you need and get out.

Your Ally in Crisis – Medical Care

*"'Don't ask questions' might be good for the
military, but it's not good in life."*

One moment Mark was running on a treadmill, preparing for his upcoming elk hunt. The next minute he was on the ground looking up at EMTs who kept him alive. Mark was in a crisis. The System, in particular the conventional medical model, is great at crisis care. Mark is alive because of the swift action of the medical technicians, the attending emergency room doctors and nurses, the medication and the surgical intervention of placing a stent in the arteries of his heart. These are the modern medicine miracles.

Crisis care keeps people alive to see another elk hunt, another day at their job, another day with their wives. Conventional medical care is great at crisis care. If you fall off your garage roof, and break a rib that punctures your lung, a medical team will save your life. If you have diabetes, insulin will save your life from being cut short by a diabetic coma. If your heart is full of plaque that is cutting off the heart's own supply of blood, a cardiac stent will save your life.

Once the crisis is done, and the long process of healing begins, you will feel gratitude for the intervention. And you should be grateful that we live in a time where a fall from a ladder doesn't end your life. Once you have been released on good behavior from the POW camp, Mission You is back on. Keep that gratitude in your heart, as it's good for healing. All gratitude is good. Millions of people in conventional medicine, from researchers to physicians to pharmacists, have dedicated *their* lives to preserving *yours* when crisis hits. Be grateful. Now back to the mission.

Mission You: Take Action

- Print from www.DrNancyTrimboli.com *The Four Medical Testing Questions*. Be prepared with this print-out at every medical appointment because recommendations for testing can be made at any time. Make notes as soon as possible.

- Continue to ask: **What if I Could Heal? Why? Where are my Resources?**

Chapter 5

FIVE REASONS TO USE MEDICATION

You are already on the first steps of your mission, Mission You. You are asking better questions: **What if I Could Heal? Why? Where are my Resources?**

You now know that you have more power than you realized. Your awareness that The System is constantly trying to regain its hold on you is a battle won. That crazy television commercial with the two people in bathtubs in a field is goofy enough to draw your attention. The movie you watched with the kids on Saturday night prominently shows the soda pop can on the leading actor's kitchen counter. Your favorite magazine now seems to be riddled with enticements to lure you to make bad food choices. Knowing that The System and its components are always vying for your attention means that you are wary of its influence.

One of the ways The System beguiles us is through medications. Medications work. Most of the time, the action of the drug fulfills its intended purpose. A symptom can be suppressed. Take the pain reliever and your headache goes away, take the little purple pill and the heartburn recedes. After three months on the statin drug the numbers become smaller on the blood test results.

Introduction into the drug system starts early in life. Toddlers and infants are put on antibiotics that clear up ear infection, antacids are used for reflux. Middle school and high school kids learn to ask Mom for medication. What should be used as a temporary crutch becomes a knee-jerk reaction to subdue a recurring symptom. Never mind about true healing.

Here is where you will exercise your new power. You've learned about your body and your problem. You can also learn about the benefits and downfalls of medications. Using the most current available data, you can choose when to take or not to take medications, at your own discretion. You are not a slave to The System any longer.

The History of Modern Medications

The System has developed medications over the last century that save us when our lives are in jeopardy. This is how The System started to gain popularity.

Before the age of antibiotics, simple infections would kill you. Imagine the horror of watching a child die from a simple injury or bacterial pneumonia, scarlet fever, or tuberculosis. After antibiotics were in use, the survival rate of children rose and the chances of dying from infection plummeted. It was miraculous. Antibiotics enhanced the effectiveness of the care medical doctors offered and elevated their position in society. The public put a lot of trust into medical doctors who not only wrote the prescriptions for the antibiotic, but in the early days dispensed the medication too. The amazing properties of antibiotics propelled human advancement.

The System also developed vaccines which appear to have eradicated childhood and adult diseases that otherwise would have killed you or created a life of infirmity. The controversy still exists as to whether these specific diseases were already on the decline because of better sewage systems and hygiene at the moment the vaccines were introduced. Even so, the medical doctor and "modern medicine" was given credit for the achievement. Each time a new drug arrived on the scene and was linked to a change in human mortality, whether deserved or not, it strengthened The System.

Medications are not all bad. It is the overuse of medication that is bad. It is the shunning of other viable, effective, and extremely safe non-drug options that is bad. It may seem like conventional medicine is beginning to embrace nondrug alternative healing arts, even so far as to call it "complementary," but an undercurrent that the nondrug healers are quacks and unscientific still exists. The discriminatory attitude which relegates the practitioners of alternative healing arts to second-class citizens has occurred since the dawn of 'modern medicine' as we know it today.

In 1910, John D. Rockefeller was a billionaire and the richest man in the world.[67] He created his wealth by becoming a magnate of oil production, and eventually owned 90% of the oil wells and pipelines in the country. The research and development for uses of petroleum by-products and petrochemicals had given us plastics in 1907, called Bakelite. It could be mass produced and was used to insulate wires for the burgeoning need for household electricity. Obviously, Rockefeller was a savvy businessman. Insulating wires was just the beginning. Medications could now be formulated from petroleum by-products into a pill, then standardized.[68] Previously, drugs were compounded by individual pharmacists and medical doctors. Aspirin, formerly sold as a powder distributed by medical doctors, became a pill in 1915.[69] Consumers could now buy it over the counter in a convenient form.

Prior to 1910, there were 155 medical schools teaching all facets of the healing arts with no standardization. Each school was different from the other. Depending on the school attended, students could learn everything from naturopathy, to homeopathy, to medical practice as it was taught in the European medical schools. Some students were taught the use of the newly discovered drugs which included cocaine and opiates.

The Flexner Report, published in 1910, subsidized by John D. Rockefeller's billions, was an exhaustive study of existing medical schools. In Rockefeller's thinking, there were too many. Those healing arts using plant-based medicine were undesirable in Rockefeller's plans. He wanted to optimize his use of petroleum by-products. Because naturopathy and homeopathy utilized plants found in nature, and not laboratory-created

---

67 History.com editors, "John D. Rockefeller," History.com, April 9, 2010, updated June 6, 2019. Accessed August 22, 2019. https://www.history.com/topics/early-20th-century-us/john-d-rockefeller.

68 Kanthan, Chris, "How Rockefeller Founded Modern Medicine and Killed Natural Cures," *World Affairs*, October 20, 2015. Accessed September 1, 2019. https://worldaffairs.blog/tag/rockefeller/.

69 Landau, Elizabeth, "From a tree, a 'miracle' called aspirin," CNN, December 22, 2010. Accessed August 22, 2019. http://www.cnn.com/2010/HEALTH/12/22/aspirin.history/index.html.

drugs that could be patented, Rockefeller had no use for those healing arts in his vision of what modern medicine would become. Encouraging the use of petrochemicals in an organized, standardized medical system was at the core of the medical school restructure. The Flexner Report found in its study that there were vast differences between medical schools. Some adhered to the code newly created from standards of teaching commonly used in Europe, but most did not. The number of medical schools in the United States was reduced from 155 to just 31. Anything related to home-opathy, naturopathy, botany, acupuncture, or chiropractic was deemed substandard and "quackery."[70] First, John D. Rockefeller had found a way to create income from his pharmaceutical by-products. He then created the consumer pipeline he needed to sell these pharmaceuticals via the medical professional. He was able to successfully shun the remainder of the safe, effective, and cheaper healing arts by first not recognizing them to be in the medical field, and then to label them as quackery.

The Spanish Flu epidemic of 1917-1918 sickened hundreds of thou-sands and killed thousands. Chiropractic was in its fledgling years with the first school, Palmer Chiropractic School, having just opened in 1897. By 1917, only six states had enacted licensure.[71] Chiropractors across the United States are reported to have been the reason why many people sur-vived rather than succumbing to the flu. In New York City, of every 10,000 cases *medically* treated, 950 people died. (That's almost a ten percent death rate.) For every 10,000 cases of the flu treated with chiropractic, only 25 patients died. (That's only one quarter of one percent.) Chiropractors in Oklahoma were sent the medical failures, people deemed lost causes and abandoned by medical doctors. Of those 233 people, all survived except for 25. That is a success rate of 89% for people that were expected to die imminently. City after city reported that the chiropractic patients survived better than the medical cases.[72]

70 Wikipedia contributors, "Flexner Report," In *Wikipedia, The Free Encyclopedia*, Accessed September 1, 2018. https://en.wikipedia.org/wiki/Flexner_Report.

71 Palmer College of Chiropractic, "History." Accessed August 22, 2019. http://www.palmer.edu/about-us/history/palmer-family.

72 Rhodes, Walter, "The Official History of Chiropractic in Texas," (Texas Chiropractic Association: 1978) Accessed November 10, 2018. https://www.danmurphydc.com/Rhodes_Flu.pdf.

It is said that because of the help chiropractors offered to the Spanish flu victims, the licensure for chiropractic gained momentum, and states set up the necessary legislature. The road to licensure for chiropractic had not been easy, and in spite of the wonderful successes in the flu epidemic, did not become easier.

In 1906, while Robert Flexner was generating data for his report to be published in 1910, and working on Rockefeller's agenda, the first chiropractor was jailed for practicing medicine without a license. These arrests and convictions continued through the 1920s and 1930s, with some articles citing 15,000 arrests made with 3300 convictions.[73,74] Conditions were harsh while in jail and prison, and some convicted had prolonged stays lasting years in length. There is a story of an individual who never recovered from the work camp and died upon release.[75] In one year, of the 600 practicing chiropractors in California at that time, 450 were arrested. The System was being formed, and holistic care was not part of it.

Prior to the Flexner Report when medicine was a non-structured healing art, homeopathy was practiced by over 30% of the then medical doctors. After the release of the report and its implementation, homeopaths were now on the outside of the new standardized medical system. They were ostracized. With infighting occurring within the field of homeopathy, no cohesion could be created. Even though homeopathy had been a viable, safe, and effective healing art since its inception, the profession struggled to survive.

Connecting the dots tells you that conventional medicine as we know it today was formed by the findings of Robert Flexner and his recommendations to John D. Rockefeller. The standards of medical school education were created to find a use for otherwise junk leftovers from oil manufacture. Petrochemicals were used in the formulation of pharmaceutical drugs and are still used today. In our modern world, petrochemicals can be found

73 Fishbein, Morris, "The Medical War," *Chiropractors for Fair Journalism*. Accessed December 12, 2018. https://chiropractorsforfairjournalism.com/Going_to_Jail.html.

74 "Go to Jail for Chiropractic!" *Dr. Lamar's Spinal Column* (blog), November 13, 2009. Accessed December 12, 2018. https://spinalcolumnblog.com/2009/11/13/go-to-jail-for-chiropractic.

75 Kent, Christopher, "Paying the Price: Going to Jail for Chiropractic," *Dynamic Chiropractic* 30, 25. December 12, 2012. Accessed August 22, 2019.

in syringes, IV bags, tubing, replacement joints, gloves, even antibacterial soap. Derivatives of Rockefeller's oil production are everywhere medical care exists. At no point in history were holistic methods such as chiropractic, homeopathy, or naturopathy vindicated as safe and effective. The persecution still occurs today. Conventional medicine continues to see those healing arts as substandard. Millions if not billions of federal (taxpayer) dollars are funneled to academic research facilities that support the doctrines of The System. Harvard, the University of California San Francisco Campus, and the University of Wisconsin all receive over $500,000,000 (five hundred million dollars) in federal grants yearly.[76] In contrast Palmer College, the oldest chiropractic learning institution, was awarded $7 million in 2017 by the National Institutes of Health for a six-year project. The Department of Defense, in association with Palmer College, completed an eight-year study in 2019 focusing on military readiness, low back pain, and smoking cessation.[77] Although these studies have produced positive results, the grants total less than $2 million a year. At four *one-thousandths of a percent*, compared to those other universities, I can say, with confidence, that nearly no federal money is apportioned for researching holistic care.

We will all likely use medication at some point. Medication is part of our society and advancements in life-saving techniques and drugs make our lives better. It is our over-reliance on medications and the lack of knowledge of other safe, effective, alternative methods that is in question.

Five Reasons to Take Medication

There will be, at times in your life, reasons to use medication. Pharmaceuticals are not necessarily bad, if you know how to use it and use it properly. Once you are aware of The System, begin to ask better questions, and realize

76   Comen, Evan, Michael Sauter, Samuel Stebbins, and Thomas Frohich, "Universities Getting the Most Money from the Federal Government," *24/7 Wall St.*, March 22, 2017. Accessed August 15, 2019. https://247wallst.com/special-report/2017/03/22/universities-getting-the-most-money-from-the-federal-government/3.

77   Palmer College, "Active Grants and Projects," Accessed September 28, 2019. https://www.palmer.edu/research/grants-projects.

that there is opportunity for healing, you may wish to avoid medications. I applaud you for that discerning choice.

As a chiropractor, my license precludes me from prescribing medication. Nor, would I want to. The philosophy of vitalism on which I operate drives me to offer other solutions that allow the body to heal. If a referral to a medical professional for a consult and possible drug intervention is the most prudent option, I gladly do it. The intent of this chapter is to illustrate your options, and to offer real world strategies. Being a Stealth Health operative means you make choices based on information. You may need to, want to, or choose to use medication.

Reason #1 to Take Medication: Under Strict Orders from an M.D.

Mark's story is an example. He was thrust into The System because of a crisis, a heart attack.

In the weeks after his heart attack, it appeared that there were no other choices. With the conventional medical model as part of The System, someone who has a heart attack is prescribed this collection of seven drugs. For his diagnosis, these medications were the next step in the algorithm. The diagnosis was getting the treatment, not Mark.

What if *you* are under strict orders to continue a medication by a medical professional? You may have heard that stopping the medication suddenly is ill-advised.

What do you do? For one, stay on your medication. Talk to your medical professional about your plans. Be sure to speak their language. Talk about your diagnosis and your symptoms. Make sure they know you have a firm understanding that the prevention of a second heart attack, or the suppression of your cough, or finding the source of the ongoing bladder infections is important. Relay in *their* language your progress. This may be with test results or symptom tracking. In Mark's case, he would monitor his blood pressure daily and write down the results. He was able to share his log of blood pressure results with his doctor at regularly scheduled visits and illustrate that removing the meds was a good choice.

You may have symptoms for which you can keep a log. If you are controlling your asthma with an alternative method, offer symptom updates, for example that you are able to sleep four hours at a time instead of two hours at a time. Or that you used your inhaler once daily for the last month rather than three times daily. Your medical professional has been trained to keep track of signs and symptoms in a quantitative fashion. Simply saying that you 'feel better' will not satisfy them or allow them to be compliant with documenting your progress.

Besides your well-being, your medical professional has a legal liability for your care, and a separate legal responsibility for documentation of your ongoing progress. At some past medical appointments, it may have seemed that your adequate completion of paperwork had more relevance than the interaction you had with the doctor. This is due to the documentation requirements, and it is separate from any malpractice liability. Failure to properly document carries with it the threat of fines and prosecution imposed by federal agencies.[78]

If you plan to use medical testing to keep track of your progress, but you are wanting to step outside of The System, be upfront with your medical professional that recommends the meds and the testing. Let them know that is your plan. Discuss with your MD the desire to reduce your medication number and dosage. Your medical professional may be able to assist you on your quest to reduce meds and tell you which tests would be most helpful to monitor yourself.

For instance, if your concern is osteoporosis (-*osteo* meaning bone, -*poros* meaning pores or holes) it may be recommended after a bone density test to take a medication. You know you don't want to risk the side effects of it, and you already have a strategy. Never mind telling your medical professional that with the nutritional program, exercise, and the bioidentical hormone replacement, you are hoping to reverse the bone thinning found on your bone density test. Unless they, like you, have heard the medication

---

78   U.S. Department of Health and Human Services. Office of Inspector General. *A Roadmap for New Physicians: Avoiding Medicare and Medicaid Fraud and Abuse.* https://oig.hhs.gov/compliance/physician-education/roadmap_web_version.pdf.

builds weakened bone after three years and are also interested in alternative options, they may not understand. Either way let your medical professional know that you will need help to monitor your progress by having a referral made for bone density tests twice per year. Speak their language by knowing more about your family history and what that means to you with your current situation. Saying things like, "Since my sister had breast cancer (of a certain type), I know that I need to be wary of soy products and get my regular mammograms," will go a long way when you wish to put off a mammogram for another year. Knowing that your sister's cancer was slow growing and knowing your doctor, above all, has concern about you will put you in the right frame of mind.

Be knowledgeable about how your personal history plays a part, and your doctor will see that your decisions are based on understanding, not just generalities. You want to make your doctor aware that you are trying to reduce the amount of toxins and trauma to your body in the way of medications and invasive testing. It's not that you are rejecting everything and anything outright.

In Mark's instance, he found that he had a medical professional that was unwilling or unable to work with him to change his medications. Mark made the choice to switch doctors. He was on seven medications and not feeling the love of life as he once had. He couldn't go on like that. When he questioned his prescribing doctor about it, no avenues of exploration to reduce his meds were forthcoming. Luckily Mark has a resource in his healthcare arsenal, a family doctor who was able to refer him to an open-minded cardiologist. His family doctor also recommended a book written by a cardiologist that helped him to understand his heart, his heart condition, and better alternatives to the medications. You can find this book and others in the resources tab on my website at www.DrNancyTrimboli.com.

Reason #2 to Take Medication: It's Your Best Bet

In this instance, you've done your homework. Although your doctors may know a lot about you, you are the expert on you. You understand how your past, meaning your family history and personal history, affect your present health issues. You have a firm grasp on the future outcome you seek. The treatment options you face are wrought with pros and cons. The best option for you may be the medical route. Drugs and/or surgery are the best option. Once you agree to and take the conventional medical route, the onus is placed on you to generate your inborn repair mechanisms. The pursuit of healing does not stop, and it is crucial after medical intervention. You are fully aware of this responsibility when you act as your own health advocate.

Certain types of cancers can respond extremely well to conventional medical treatment. As we all know, treatment for cancer that aims to destroy the cancer cells can also destroy your body. Once you undertake that as your treatment, tapping into your healthcare resources is essential to thrive after the treatment. If you choose this path, you will become an expert on supporting your body as it is being broken down and rebuilt.

Another example is acute Lyme disease. Generally, antibiotics should be avoided whenever possible. In the case of Lyme disease, specific antibiotics have been demonstrated to greatly reduce long-term effects of the infection. However, antibiotic use, especially the strong antibiotics used for Lyme disease, will destroy the natural flora of the gut. If prebiotics and probiotics are not used, severe intestinal problems will ensue. You must take over your own self-care. Whether your medical doctor recommends probiotics or not, you likely need to do your own research and use it.

Genetic abnormalities which would have killed a person as a child born a century ago now can be controlled with drugs. One such disorder is blood that clots too easily. Using a blood thinner throughout this person's life will allow them to be fully functional although they may need to be wary of foods or medications that have a blood thinning effect. In all cases, supporting your body through nutrition, chiropractic, homeopathy, acupuncture, bodywork, and other methods will enhance your body's ability to heal. Do all your homework when faced with decisions like these. Continue to investigate as you go through treatment and especially if you need ongoing medical care throughout your life. Ask the powerful questions, keep your resources close, and follow leads to new healing paths.

Reason #3 to Take Medication: It's Right for Right Now

Mentally, you are ready for the mystery to unfold. Your body, however, is tired. Your symptoms from your issues drag you down. Using a medication can help you through your busy days and keep symptoms in check while you investigate your leads, assemble your healthcare arsenal of people, and give holistic methods a chance to work. Just because you are engaged in a Stealth Health mission doesn't mean you must reject the symptom relief you've used thus far. Please don't see this as a sign of defeat. It's a stepping-stone. You are using the best that conventional medicine has to offer with knowledge and careful consideration.

For example, thyroid problems can result in a lack of energy, sleeplessness, feelings of weakness and being cold. Until the underlying cause, the **Why?** is discerned, using thyroid medication can alleviate some of these symptoms.

Theresa's Tricky Thyroid

Theresa had more energy than she'd had in a long time and, based on that, thought the thyroid levels on her blood test would come back normal. But the T3, T4, and thyroid antibody levels looked the same as the previous test done three months ago.

"I feel better, though," she said to Dr. Martin, her general practitioner.

Theresa didn't want to stay on the thyroid drugs. She'd always been so diligent to take care of herself, and this seemed like she was admitting defeat. What would be next… Increasing the dosage? Removing her thyroid? She had read some books about nutritional health for the thyroid, and she didn't want to mention it to Dr. Martin. She didn't know what kind of reaction she'd receive from him. Mention it and risk pushback, like "stop reading books."

Little did Theresa know that in two weeks she would be bitten by a tick carrying Lyme disease. The pain was uncontrolled by any narcotic, the fatigue debilitating. Just because of the sheer exhaustion, she stopped taking all her medications, all of her vitamins. She struggled just to feed herself.

The illness dragged on even after the heavy-duty antibiotics given during her hospital stay. For the pain, acupuncture and Chinese herbs was the answer. Although the infectious disease doctor considered her cured, she believed she was far from that. The foggy, confused thinking and the skin rashes told her otherwise. She recalled a holistic health-care professional who specialized in Lyme disease. The electromagnetic testing indicated severe organ malfunction. The regimen of homeopathic remedies and supplements took her 45 minutes each day to organize. A big part of the reason for the severity of her Lyme disease was an underlying weakness in her liver that had gone undetected on previous routine medical blood tests. After thirty days with the holistic remedies, she was showing improvement, and continued taking it. After six months, she returned to Dr. Martin for a regularly scheduled exam on her thyroid. This time, the thyroid test was normal. Fixing her liver had fixed her thyroid.

I would never suggest that succumbing to a disease as destructive as Lyme is a way to solve any mission. Nor, that homeopathy is a panacea for thyroid issues. The most pervasive diseases in our society are that way for a reason. Osteoporosis, hyperthyroidism, hypothyroidism, infertility, digestive trouble, and cardiac problems are difficult to solve or manage because they are multifactorial and likely stem from discord throughout the body. When choosing a holistic path which improves function overall, healing can and will occur from sources known, and from the deep mysterious healing capabilities we all possess. As you manage your everyday life with medication, embark on your mission to rebuild from the inside out.

Super-sized Pain

Brian was a big human: a full-on, supersize, take-it-to-the-max kind of guy. That fact plus his love of playing football and years of high-wire acts while heaving rebar as an ironworker caused him to need a hip replacement at age 48. And that's without mentioning the snowmobile, car, and motocross accidents. Before he agreed to go under the knife, a mishap from his lack of mobility caused him to suffer greater damage.

Falling off a twenty-foot-high hunting platform stopped him in his tracks like nothing ever had. To repair the seven fractures of his leg, the surgery was estimated to take seven hours. The surgical team worked on him for twelve hours. He wouldn't walk for months, and his recovery would require large amounts of opioid medication to be able to tolerate the pain, just to take the edge off.

After three months, he decided to taper down. "Of course, I can," he thought, and attempted to accelerate the taper down process. After all, everything he did was more direct than anyone else. When the cold sweats and trembling started, he realized the hold that the drugs had on him. Over time, he cut down the pills very slowly as the pharmacist told him to do. After twenty days when he held the dust from an eighth of a pill in his fingertips, he knew he had beaten it.

Necessary Pain Medication

Drugs that are essential for managing the pain from a surgery or an injury can also lead to addiction. Immediately after the surgery or injury, follow the recommendation of your medical professional, which may include opioid drugs. Having a plan in place to reduce the dependence on the drug over time is imperative. Use those people in your healthcare arsenal to understand the pain and utilize bodywork and nondrug remedies to manage the pain as you heal. Until different nonaddictive methods for postsurgical, postinjury pain are in widespread use, this is our best option.

Sad to Sadder

Tanya, who was unhappy with her job when her boss passed her up for a promotion, was also not getting along with her husband. She didn't consider other options or look up the side effects before starting the anti-anxiety medication.

After two months she wished that she had investigated first. The medication had stopped the panic attacks but replaced it with feelings of despair and fatigue. Recently she started to wake in a sweat, with a sense of fear that she had never felt before. Her repeated calls and visits to the medical practice that had prescribed her the meds responded with a suggestion to see a psychologist. It was her pharmacist that explained to her how to wean herself from the medication.

She told me, "I don't know what to do. The night terrors make me afraid to lie down at night. My moods are worse than before."

In Tanya's case she had to stay on the medication even with the side effects so that she could slowly reduce her dosage. Now, after having read a book on brain health, she is juicing every day and noticed a big shift in her ability to cope with her anxiety and depression after just one week. Her improved mood has helped her relationship with her husband. Her job is still the same, but now, she's content with it.

Investigate Before You Take

You may be one of the millions battling anxiety and depression. Do what is necessary to protect yourself and those you love while actively looking for answers. One of the most memorable direct-to-consumer-marketing advertisements of 2001 featured sad balloons that became happy by the end of the thirty-second television spot.[79] Based on the sales of this drug (which in 2001 topped $2.3 billion),[80] the commercial obviously motivated people to ask for this drug by name for their panic attacks or depression. Many may have been recommended to take it by their doctor. Unfortunately, some antianxiety medications lead to, ironically, anxiety as a side effect. Suicidal thoughts and actions are also a serious side effect. If anyone is considering a drug of this type, consulting www.askapatient.com would give them some insight.

---

79 "Original Zoloft Commercial." *YouTube*. March 12, 2009. Accessed July 18, 2019. https://www.youtube.com/watch?v=twhvtzd6gXA.

80 "Pfizer Bucks Pharma Trend," *CNN Money*, December 18, 2001. Accessed July 27, 2019. https://money.cnn.com/2001/12/18/companies/pfizer/index.htm.

Reason #4 to Take Medication: The One and Done

Sometimes you have to be more like MacGyver. If you never watched that TV show, all you really need to know is that he used everyday objects to get himself out of jams. At times you will need to MacGyver a fix so that you can get away from a symptom. This particular symptom is short lived. "Self-limiting" is what your medical professional would call it. It's not a symptom that plagues you. You can use the raw materials around you, or from your friendly neighborhood drug store, to patch together a fix.

For these issues, you might know the cause, or maybe not. In the future, the likelihood of staying on this drug is low. Perhaps right now you only need to know how to stop the symptoms. The **Why?** is elusive. More than likely it's a temporary problem that will fix itself. One thing is for sure; you have a symptom that needs a fix right now. No delay. Right now. Knowing the actions of medications will help you use some over-the-counter drugs for immediate relief of various symptoms. Keep an armory of medication at the ready for common issues.

Imagine you are about to board a plane with your family for a Florida spring break vacation. Your ten-year-old son announces as he emerges from the men's room that he's got diarrhea. You've got your portable armory at the ready. You give him a digestive medication that will get all of you through the flight.

Or maybe you have seasonal allergies. If you've ever been in Georgia in the springtime, you've seen the yellow dust that covers everything: cars, parking lots, your coffee table if you leave the patio door open. This dust also covers your sinus cavities and can cause allergic responses in some people. Using an over-the-counter antihistamine will reduce your body's response to the pollen when you go to the Peachtree Conference Center in April.

Then there is the self-inflicted trauma. This comes in many forms. Typically, it results in inflammation of some type. It could be the pesky lower back disc that you inflame when you help your neighbor move the ancient television out of the basement. Maybe it's those sourdough rolls at the best restaurant in Toledo that you know will trigger your thumb joints to swell. But you eat it anyway, because you love it. Or the time when your best friend forgets your food sensitivity to eggs when she makes you a birthday cake. Over-the-counter anti-inflammatories to the rescue. As much as we beat ourselves up, and promise to be extra careful in the future, plan on using meds to assist you.

In these cases, you take medication for a very short-term physiological reason. You have empowered yourself with knowledge on how they work. Using these drugs to your advantage, you are aware that they may add value to your life in the immediate future. But you aren't a chronic user. These are one-offs; individual opportunities to use the vast resources of The System to your advantage.

Reason #5 to Take Medication: A (Truly) Permanent Condition

In this case you take medication because of a physical limitation of matter. A physical limitation of matter means that you have a permanent condition. Some cells of your body or some organ of your body is now nonfunctional.

This could be due to your genetics. For example, you may be diagnosed with type 1 diabetes early in life. You may never go off insulin. In this case, lifelong insulin will maintain your quality of life.

Or, it could be that an injury, a fall, or a car accident changed your body in ways to render it not fixable. The body repairs with scar tissue. Sometimes scar tissue traps a tiny nerve that causes a persistent pain. Structural imbalances due to those injuries could now affect how you walk, move, sit, or lay, which may be improved but never corrected.

Surgeries change us forever. Before you embarked on this Stealth Health journey of regaining true wellness, it is possible that you have had an organ removed. A medical professional didn't stop to ask, "**Why** do many forty-year-old, overweight females have gallbladder problems?" The recommendation was made to remove your gallbladder, and you did it. You may have developed goiters in you thyroid, and, instead of asking **What if I Could Heal?**, you had your thyroid irradiated.

Previous lifestyle choices, cigarette smoking, excessive drinking, or drug use, may have led to organ disease, and continued neglect has rendered it malfunctional. The damage has led to lifelong challenges.

You also could have had a crisis in your past which caused you to choose a path to medication which has left you with some permanent damage. For example, simple but distracting joint pain can lead many to overuse anti-inflammatory drugs to the point of stomach ulcers.

You may be dealing with PTSD which has left you with emotional scars, but you're able to live life near normally with psychiatric medication. You could have been diagnosed with an inoperable brain tumor, and the seizures it causes can be controlled with medication.

These changes to your body and choices made in the past now cause you to disclose this weakness at every new health practitioner appointment. You are labeled. You feel like damaged goods. Even with that being the case, never shut down the possibility for change, as Hector's story illustrates.

(Not) A Permanent Disability

"I have weakness in my legs because of my M.S. That's what my doctor told me," Hector said to me during his new patient consultation. (M.S. stands for multiple sclerosis, a diagnosis for a condition in which the protective fatty covering of the central nervous system neurons is destroyed.)

"My balance problems, too. I don't expect you to help me with that. I'm here because my lower back hurts me. I can't sit for longer than 30 minutes before I have to shift my hips to one side. I spend a lot of time in my recliner."

He told me this as I was examining him, checking the strength of his leg muscles as I always do, on everyone. Hector had come to me for chiropractic care for his lower back pain on the recommendation of his mother.

I didn't mention that the chiropractic adjustments we would do for his lower back pain might also help his leg strength and the balance issues. Or maybe I did. Either way, he would not have believed me. He wouldn't have believed me because his doctor had given him a reason for the leg weakness. He gave Hector a label of M.S. that covers a lot of bases: pain, weakness, and balance problems.

After our twelve-visit treatment plan, he filled out his assessment questionnaire. He wrote: "Back is 100% better. Played pool with the boys last night for 2 hours! I haven't been able to stand for that long or play pool like that in years!" On examination, his legs were strong, and his balance was perfect. He had believed the limits that his medical professional had given him, and never sought an answer to his weakness, pain, and unsteadiness. He believed that he was at his optimum. He wasn't. Simple chiropractic adjustments gave him a new optimum.

No matter what the scenario, you still can make changes and heal. There may be limitations for you that others do not have. Your optimal health level may not be what it once was. Almost certainly if you follow a healing path, if you start and continue to uncover clues and follow the leads, you will unravel your mystery. Just like Jason Bourne can never have his old life back, or even remember his old life, your limitations are there. Those exist. But, also just like Jason Bourne, you can expand your understanding of yourself. You can learn how your body works and use this new knowledge and power to live a fuller life. You can do it. You can make changes if you take the steps.

You Call the Shots

Using medications to your advantage is a way to use resources inside of The System without relinquishing complete control. Being conscious of the judicial use of medication is the next step to take back your power and solve Mission You. Consciously taking medication for reasons that have been predetermined by you keeps you one step ahead of The System. When you open that pill bottle, you are like our spy hero opening the door to step into the game room of the tycoon whose heavyweight-champion-like bodyguards are waiting to take you down. But you have stealth on your side, you have your own best interest on your side, and you know what you are looking for in that trophy room. You can see the bodyguards looking in the opposite direction. You are there for a reason. You are in control of your every move, no one else. With your powerful questions in mind of **What if I Could Heal?**, **Why?**, and **Where are my Resources?**, you know that medication can be a means to an end. An end that is in sight, with you controlling what occurs from here to there in Mission You.

Mission You: Take Action

- Make a list of your current medications both over-the-counter and prescription. Have you been labeled with a diagnosis that has closed the door to exploring better options? Do you have permanent limitations (removal of a limb or an organ, or verified genetic abnormality) that truly require you to be on a medication for the rest of your life? What if that's not true?

- Do you have an armory of medications that you utilize for short-lived scenarios mentioned above?

- Or do those "one-off" scenarios happen over and over? Perhaps there is an underlying issue that you are masking with medication.

- Do you possess other options in your armory that are *not* medications? Have you researched essential oils that are effective for many short-term issues? Do you have supplements to use when needed to address some of the examples listed above? If not, start a plan to accumulate these alternative methods. Expanding your knowledge will edge you one step further from The System's influence over you.

Chapter 6

THREE SOURCES TO TRUST, AND THREE TO BEWARE

YOU ARE ON the first steps of Mission You. While putting the pieces together is hard work, you will find that small steps over time create momentum. Ask better questions, and doorways of opportunity open. Whole professions with new avenues for healing are discovered that were unknown to you previously. Managing yourself becomes easier, yet there are possibly still times when your health condition runs your life. It may be slow, steady improvement, or ups and downs with relapses for no apparent reason. Even so, there is improvement. Healing changes *are* taking place.

Family and friends that have watched you suffer may not understand the timeline of healing. In our society today, we are conditioned to immediacy. We drive up to one window and get breakfast in sixty seconds. We drive up to another window and get three hundred dollars in thirty seconds. Our life is automated and fast. Our human bodies, however, are still the model built two million years ago. Human biology changes slowly. Overnight miracles can occur, but that is rare. Miracles are the exception to the rule. Healing takes time. Be patient with yourself. Celebrate your successes.

Source to Trust #1:
A Proven Holistic Healthcare Practitioner

You are unraveling the truth. To identify your true allies, and to be aware of false friends, is key. As you assemble the people in your resources, (your healthcare arsenal), you'll need to be on the lookout for new members. The good news is that birds of a feather flock together. One good resource will very likely lead you to more.

True Healing

Robert began searching for answers. He had digestive issues that were becoming worse, and the stress from his job as an air traffic controller accentuated the urgency to fix it. He had been to his primary care doctor who set him up with a barrage of tests, followed by treatment with antibiotics. Robert grew worse. He was sent to a gastrointestinal specialist who, in turn, referred him to an infectious disease doctor. They put Robert through the ringer with more tests, more medication, now for parasites. He felt hopeful at first. His body didn't feel as heavy and his digestion was better. Then he worsened again. When the infectious disease doctor recommended more meds, Robert asked me if I had any other ideas. He listened to my suggestion, consulted with the naturopath, and stayed true to the remedies suggested. Today, he has holistic care to thank for the increased energy and stamina.

"The medical profession wants to give you a Band-Aid, but holistic remedies have true healing," he said when I asked him for an update. The indigestion and problems with elimination that stumped his medical doctors were nearly resolved. And, he was free from medication. Like Robert, you will need someone on your side who is a holistic healthcare professional.

They are fully aware of the faults of The System and can be your greatest ally. There is a world of opportunity for health and healing, and many times those resources are right outside your back door. Perhaps not literally but certainly in your town, city, or county. It may be a massage therapist, your chiropractor, or a homeopath. It could be a trusted relative or friend who is a Feldenkrais practitioner, a functional medicine doctor, or a bio-reso-nance practitioner. Don't discount medical professionals either. Every day, medical doctors who have, up to now, practiced conventional medicine, see the weaknesses of it. They set out to become self-made experts on alternative avenues for healing. Do you remember Mark from Chapter 2? His introduction to learning about his heart issue came from his general practitioner who has made such a transition. His doctor told him, "My favorite surgery is a pill-ectomy." We should all be so lucky to have a person like him in our arsenal.

I cannot say that there is consistency, and that *every* practitioner who is under the general heading of holistic has a similar viewpoint. It sounds contradictory, I know. As a general rule, you will find holistic practitioners are open to new ideas, new paradigms, and are not afraid to eschew standard conventional medical practices. Conventional medical practices have left us in the mess that we are in. Most holistic practitioners are not afraid to recognize that. Choose one with whom you share viewpoints.

There are multiple reasons to use a holistic provider as your go-to source. My patients, both current and former, know that they can ask me an array of questions. Recent questions I've received are: What do you know about Meridian Stress Tests? (A little bit.) Any recommendations for low testosterone? (Yes.) My mom fell, she's fine, no fractures, does she need to be adjusted? (Yes.) My friend says she isn't feeling well, right arm went numb, then right side of her mouth … and she's tired. Is that an emergency? (Yes! Go to the ER!) My daughter leaves for college in a few weeks. Can you recommend a chiropractor for her? (Yes.)

As holistic practitioners, we have our finger on the pulse of new ideas and influence from thought leaders across genres. Our alternative ideas, and the array of books, people, and websites in our own personal arsenal can assist you in the unraveling of your mystery. Things like earthing, shungite stones, muscle testing to know which supplements are correct in the moment, the use of biosensors, tapping, magnet therapy, hair mineral analysis testing, and a gaggle of other apparatus and ideas are within our knowledge base as practitioners. Yet holistic remedies and techniques vary greatly. Just because I know a world of information about chiropractic doesn't mean that I know a hoot about naturopathy. I hope to increase my knowledge base, and yours, of these different approaches by personally interviewing experts and bringing the details to you. Check my website for that intel.

So many opportunities for healing exist that no one person can be an expert on everything, or even have been introduced to it all. Since holistic providers know each other, if one of us doesn't know an answer, a simple phone call can fix that. Not only are these providers aware of each other, they likely have shared services. Portions of their arsenal may become parts of yours. For me, I use acupuncture, massage therapy, colon therapy, CranioSacral therapy, lymphatic drainage, bioidentical hormone therapy, and energy medicine routinely. As our patients begin to broaden their inclination for holistic healing, we may send them to someone in our own arsenal. For instance, an acupuncturist and a chiropractor have an overlap of patients who use the services of both. We aren't in competition with each other; on the contrary, we work in conjunction with each other.

As you speak to your new health practitioners about your desires to heal and to free yourself of processed foods, medications and dead-end diagnoses, they may reveal paths for you to explore. Use their knowledge, use their expertise, use their connections, take recommendations on books, and explore the next steps on your own to investigate. Follow through on their advice.

A good timeframe to know if a treatment will work is at least two weeks, but preferably six weeks. That is contingent upon your compliance with the treatment recommendations. In my office, if I tell someone that I need to see them twelve times within six weeks to see lasting and significant improvement and they've only walked through my door twice in six weeks, we likely will not meet our goals. Once you commit to a treatment plan, carve the time, energy, and money out of your life to make it happen. Walking through my door can be the hardest part, I know. Make yourself the priority in Mission You.

When you've taken the next step on your path, let your health provider know. For me, that's what is most fulfilling—seeing you regain your life, unravel your mystery, and break free of The System.

Regarding payment for holistic practitioners, whatever money you dole out is worth multiple magnitudes back in value. This stuff works. You would think that insurance companies would want to support safer, more effective, and less expensive strategies for improving health. With some policies, decreased premiums are offered for lower body mass index, nonsmokers, and sometimes for workplace exercise facilities. However, the insurance industry was trained in the ways of The System. Conventional medicine does not understand vitalistic avenues, therefore insurance providers don't either. If you have insurance benefits for chiropractic or acupuncture, try to use the benefits. But, and I say this with a sigh and a knowing nod, years of experience in the health insurance arena as an in-network healthcare provider, as an insured with my own health benefits, and as an employer attempting to procure insurance coverage for my staff, it ain't all sunshine and roses. Be prepared to pay cash money (or credit card or checks) for the best care.

For some, and this depends on the rules of your specific plan, the Health Savings Account (HSA) is a way to pay for care that is outside of your insurance benefits. If you have a large deductible with an HSA to augment your plan, ask your administrator.

In my experience, people are so satisfied (and at times, amazed) with their vitalistic and holistic practitioners that they gladly pay out of pocket. When results are real, and not merely symptom suppression with medication, you will do so as well.

Source to Trust #2:
Books, Documentaries, Podcasts, Websites and Internet Searches

Seen on a poster in a local pet store: Photo of a dog's golden-furred right front leg on which a medical bracelet has the following: "The internet says I either have tennis elbow, or hitchhiker's thumb, or the black plague."

Yes, the internet can be a minefield. Seriously, this topic could be in both the "who to trust" and the "who to beware" sections. I'll make it easy for you: Trusted authors of books, directors of documentaries, and hosts of podcasts *lead to* authorities with their own websites *lead to* other helpful websites, podcasts and books. *In that order.*

In previous years, you could jump in and do an internet search and find good results. But The System has gotten a hold of the first page of searches. Try this and you'll see for yourself. Search for "holistic care for _____" or "natural cures for _____" or "nondrug approach for _____." You'll have to do some rummaging through domains to find ones that have genuine, not slanted information. Look out for an obvious, or not so obvious, attempt by The System to hook you right back to the same old rhetoric (an obvious conventional medical site), or a page with simplistic but lame remedies (in my opinion) that could lead to failure, or you could possibly find a gem amongst the rubble. I find that first typing my query into the text box to be fruitless unless I'm willing to sort through the second and third pages of the search. Which I have done, but with minimal success.

The best way to find great health leads is to start with books. I find new book titles from citations or endorsements in current books that I am reading. These are quotes of praise in the first few pages from other supportive authors. I've also found great leads from, not traditional magazines, but airline magazine articles. It seems like an odd place but remember that much of the media, including the written content of mainstream magazines, is controlled by advertisers. And the most lucrative advertisers are the drug industry. *Heavy sigh. This gets dull after a while, I know.* But, airline magazine advertisers are not pill pushers. To help, I have a research library to get you started. See www.DrNancyTrimboli.com for my trusted resources.

If you choose to jump into the rummage sale of internet searches, be stealthy. Websites do not adhere to the type of professional journalistic integrity rules that books do. Therefore, because you read something online does not make it true. At the same time, because you read it online does not make it *not* true. Cross-check the information on one website by looking at the end of the article for footnotes. These will lead to the originating articles or expert quotes used by the author of the article. Or, in the body of the text there may be a mention of the expert or book. By reading the source articles, you can confirm information and find clarity. It's sort of like that term paper you did in seventh grade in which you researched the gross domestic product of the state of California. You visited websites, collected information, documented the web addresses and wrote your paper. (For those my age or older, your research was done at the library using physical books and index cards. But it's the same idea.) Except now you are gaining insights and information about something far more interesting and useful… Mission You.

Another booby trap is "chat rooms" that were popular in previous decades. Avoid those. I've never found usable information there. Bloggers can be good or bad. Some seem to be receiving a paycheck directly from The System, but I can't be sure. YouTube videos are gaining traction in the health field. Just as with websites, check the sources, inspiration, and then make a judgment call on their ties to The System. Don't expect to find all the answers in one sitting. You are pursuing a pathway to help regain your health. It's a pathway with steppingstones, not a moving sidewalk, and you choose each step as you go. Do yourself a favor and have a way to save links of the most helpful sites on your PC or mobile device. OneNote or Evernote is a way to keep full articles with links in one place that is searchable and portable.

At times, you will notice an internet search brings up repeated verbiage as though one website exactly copied the information from another, leaving you to wonder which one came first, and if the content is trustworthy. Years ago, automated programs, called bots, searched the internet for a topic, and through a process called web scraping duplicated the information. After a series of legal cases, this practice is now monitored and penalized by search engines. Websites mirroring identical information still exist today. It may be good information, but it's redundant.[81]

With the internet, podcasts, and books, you can hear and see the words of others with similar issues. The health explorers of our time document their failures and successes and create content. You can learn from them through their stories. Self-made experts are created due to adversity. They may have had a sick child, or a previous illness themselves, or have tested their program on patients as a healthcare provider. The person who shares their journey of unraveling their own mystery might have a recipe for success that would help you. You can expect to learn from them. Rogue and unique information on a website doesn't necessarily make it incorrect.

81 Stemler, Sam. "Eight Ways Duplicate Content on Different Domains Hurts Ymy website." *Web Ascender*. March 8, 2018. Accessed January 15, 2020. https://www.webascender.com/blog/8-ways-duplicate-content-on-different-domains-hurts-your-website.

An abundance of guidance has been intentionally hidden from us. Simple changes can heal people quickly, while other remedies require time and complexity. Every journey is unique. Someone's own stealth health story could hold the secrets to your success.

So, yes, use the internet, do your research, investigate multiple sources, compare notes and formulate your own plan. Please, however, resist the urge to diagnose yourself. Especially don't diagnose yourself on a medical website. Avoid looking at horrible pictures or inundating yourself with worst-case scenarios. This is not helpful. You have your own drama, in your own life, and you know the unique effects of your health issue. Look for the success stories. With regards to diagnosing yourself, the only benefit to a diagnosis is to help you to explore. Naming your symptoms with a Latin name does not help. It may possibly get you sympathy at cookouts and cocktail parties, but it does nothing to help you. Calling your foot pain *plantar fasciitis* is irrelevant. If you find yourself saying, "Ahhh. That's my problem. I have irritable bowel syndrome, a neuroma of the second and third metatarsal, or ankylosing spondylitis…" Stop. Step away from the screen. Don't label yourself.

You will make discoveries and wonder what has kept this enlightenment from you and from the public in general. Like, seriously, a combination of essential oils with fennel and peppermint can be rubbed on your belly for a tummy ache?[82] That's amazingly simple… *What gives?* The System does not support and will attempt to suppress anything that is contrary to its number one agenda. Its number one agenda is to perpetuate itself. The issues you developed over your lifetime due to antibiotics, unnecessary surgery to remove organs, excess sugar, food additives, petroleum by-products, chemicals, and all the rest put you at risk. The System has no regard or remorse for its part in that. You are collateral damage. In order for The System to keep running and tricking the next generation of consumers (meaning your kids and grandkids), you must be fully committed to all it has to offer now. Fixing your health issues will extricate you from The System, and that is not on its agenda. The System does not want you to know that there is a world

---

82 www.Doterra.com/DigestZen

of opportunity for health and healing. But the joke is on them because it is literally now at our fingertips.

Look for teachers on the internet that have paved a path for you. They have been where you are right now. It is daunting and can be dangerous to be the first to forge a path in the wild unknown. They have taken risks to be one of the first so that your path will be easier to pilot. You may learn some new words along the way. You may need to learn how the body functions. You can do it. The System has taught us to be able to say and to spell *acetaminophen*. You can learn about you with no problem.

Beware of websites that are a façade of benevolent helpfulness behind which is really The System setting a trip wire. The American Heart Association (AHA) purports to have funded more research than any other organization ($4.5 billion).[83] Financial reports on the website for fiscal year 2017-2018 reveal 30 million dollars donated from pharmaceutical companies, medical device companies, and insurance companies.[84] One hundred and forty-six million came from other corporations. Reading an article on cholesterol posted on the AHA site will show you The System at work. The article recapped an old-fashioned notion that *all* fats should be restricted if faced with high cholesterol.[85] No mention was made about good fats that should be included in the diet. The idea that LDLs are "bad" was perpetuated. The biggest gaffe is the missing fact that statin drugs suppress production of coenzyme Q10 (CoQ10) in the body, and those on statin drugs should take CoQ10 as a dietary supplement. Inadequate amounts of CoQ10 starve muscles of energy with the heart muscle being the biggest consumer.[86] Old information and poor direction puts you back in the hands of The System.

83 American Heart Association. "Scientific Research," Accessed September 13, 2019. https://www.heart.org/en/about-us/scientific-research.

84 "2017-2018 American Heart Association Support from Pharmaceutical and Biotech Companies, Device Manufacturers and Health Insurance Providers," Accessed September 13, 2019. https://www.heart.org/en/about-us/aha-financial-information.

85 "Cholesterol," Accessed September 13, 2019. https://www.heart.org/en/health-topics/cholesterol.

86 Sinatra Stephen, "CoQ10 Facts: CoQ10 Benefits, Dosage & More," DrSinatra.com. Accessed September 13, 2019. https://www.drsinatra.com/coq10-facts-coq10-benefits-dosage-and-more.

There are some relevant books that existed prior to the dawn of digital content or are too complex to be used as a reference tool online. One such book is *Encyclopedia of Natural Medicine* by Michael Murray and Joseph Pizzorno. It is my go-to reference to get a handle on organ systems, the medical treatment for many disorders, and a naturopathic discussion of alternative options.[87] It's not exhaustive but it's a good place to start. As you and your fellow readers all face different struggles with a broad variety of issues, *Stealth Health* cannot attempt to teach all there is to know about each organ system, or the vast array of healing opportunities. Think of the *Stealth Health* method as a new map feature on your phone, or a spiral-bound road atlas of all fifty states. I'll show you how to use the map, but you determine your destination, your path, and the mode you'll use to get there. Capiche?

Authors of today's world have strong internet personalities to allow their audience to access free content, with additional avenues to reach the author and their expertise. I caution you with books in the same way that I caution online information. Follow the money. If a book or publication has an obvious slant supporting The System, is derogatory to whole factions of a healing art, or can be traced to a profit or nonprofit agency related to a drug company, don't trust its content. A vast array of book recommendations to help discern your path on Mission You is available at my website, www.DrNancyTrimboli.com. Additions are made regularly as I discover them.

Source to Trust #3: Unexpected Discoveries

Have you ever noticed when a friend gives you a full endorsement of a restaurant, a movie, or a book, they don't feel the need to explain it? You are having lunch with a friend discussing the latest action movie, and they say, "You just have to go." No qualifiers, no explanations, no bullet points of pros and cons. "Just go," is what they say.

Any explanation would dilute the magnificence of it. We all do this. We recognize when someone else does it. The experience was so rich it can't

---

87 Murray, Michael, and Joseph Pizzorno. *Encyclopedia of Natural Medicine*, Third Edition (New York: Atria paperback, a division of Simon & Schuster)

be described. Reducing the splendor of it to mere words would cheapen it. Only the experience itself is adequate. "Just go," they say.

When a friend or relative does this regarding healthcare, heed the advice. If the path is not right for you in the immediate future, file it away. List it on your *My Healthcare Arsenal* spreadsheet. This healthcare provider or method obviously has something special, and could, at least, be a resource for you. And notice, it didn't involve selling, cajoling, or convincing. Just sharing.

When you accepted Mission You, you thought you would be traveling it alone. You will find, however, that allies exist all around you. When you ask the right questions, ordinary encounters can bring you the answers and the people with the answers. Listen and pay attention as the information or clue to a new path of exploration will be fleeting. Be all eyes and ears and be prepared to take notes. Have a pen and your *Mission You Journal Page* at the ready.

No Selling, Just Sharing

My friend, Greg, and I were preparing for an event. It was black tie preferred, about 300 people. I was the Master of Ceremonies, and I couldn't talk because of laryngitis from a sinus infection.

Greg said, "You sound awful. Have you ever tried the sinus irrigation? No, not the little teapot thing. The pulsed water jets. It stopped my sinus infections. I use it every day still." Greg saw a friend in need and told me what helped him. He didn't ask what else I was doing, didn't tell me I was all wrong, didn't issue a warning that whatever I had tried was dangerous. I could detect no emotional investment on his part.

That was it. The one comment. The one comment that sent me to the internet to buy the water jet contraption thing. I had to figure it out for myself as Greg didn't expand on his instruction to me. I bought it, used it, and it changed my life.[88]

My questions were being answered because I was asking them. Your

88 Trimboli, Nancy. "4 Sinus Tips." *YouTube*. October 22, 2018. *https://www.youtube.com/watch?v=N79khU7hbOU*

allies are all around you too. Pay attention and continue to ask the right questions. The answers will reveal themselves.

Source to Beware #1:
A Medical Doctor That's Entwined in The System

Madeline looked like she had just been in a bar fight and lost. She is sixty years old and fell on the treadmill that afternoon, diving forward in an attempt to save herself, and dislocated her right arm and injured her left in the process. She did a faceplant on the hard plastic and metal of the treadmill, giving her a blackeye. She knew the number one place to be was the emergency room to stabilize her arm and clear her of a concussion. She called her boss, an M.D., from the ER who had one scathing remark to say about her situation. Her first stop after that—my office.

Madeline was sitting on my adjustment table with bruises all over her face, her right arm immobilized with a brace because of the shoulder dislocation, unable to lift her left arm, and her face wincing with pain at every word because of an apparent jaw misalignment.

"A bone crusher?! That's the last thing you should do." Although barely able to open her mouth, she felt it important to relay this remark from her boss, an orthopedic surgeon, when she mentioned to him that she desperately needed a chiropractic adjustment.

Only because I know her so well, I responded, "That comment set back both our professions seventy-five years. You would think he'd know better than that." She rolled her eyes knowing that his opinion, which, if directed toward someone not as savvy as her, would come across as medical advice. It had no basis in fact. It was the fiction of his own mind, as he had never experienced chiropractic for himself.

Usually when I hear the "bone crusher" label, it's from someone looking at me in the eye and grinning. If you are going to choose to become a chiropractor, you can't let jokes like that bother you. It comes with the territory. But over the years I've had patients report to me derogatory comments made by their medical doctors, either about chiropractic or other holistic healing methods. Funny thing is they fail to realize that their patient will jet it over to my office to share. Here's a small sampling of them:

"I don't know enough about it. So, don't do that."

"Whatever you do, don't see a chiropractor."

"Stop looking things up online."

"Stop reading books."

"If it helps you, keep doing it."

This last one is usually about as good as it gets when discussing alternative, or nonconventional paths with a professional inside The System. But even that is rare. More often it's one of the others.

There are exceptions to the rule. As we discussed, Mark has a gem of a doctor on his side who freely refers to other medical doctors outside The System and refers to holistic care providers, like me. Keep these members of your healthcare arsenal close. Another exception to the rule is moments when you are in a crisis situation, again like Mark. If you have a serious injury, or an acute infection, or are prone to relapses of a life-threatening illness, a medical doctor may save your life.

Crisis care is not health care, however. Treating someone for a kidney stone, a diabetic coma, or a skull fracture is essential, but a far cry from optimizing health. The problem with relying on a medical doctor for true health is that medical doctors are part of The System. They didn't intend to be. It happens all the same though. Medical professionals of all sorts end up in The System because they wanted a good job (with benefits), or their mom is a medical doctor, or they wanted to help people. Some study specific areas of medicine because it is of interest to them, or the pay is good, and they have the grades to get into that specialty. Medical students live under extreme conditions with lengthy classroom lecture time, hours of study other than the classroom, lack of good nutrition, and lack of sleep. They become suggestible. They are sponges soaking up all information whether true, conjured, or in jest.

In medical school, there is no course of study on chiropractic or acupuncture or *anything* alternative. Nutrition, even how much water to drink, or what to eat during pregnancy, is not part of the curriculum. If a medical doctor has done extensive postgraduate study in an alternative healing art, you may put trust in their opinion. Weekend seminars don't count.

You may appreciate your medical doctor, like I do mine. Your medical doctor has given you some good advice over the years and has assisted you in a variety of crises. Your medical doctor knows you. Even considering this and their friendly but authoritative demeanor, they have no knowledge about alternative healing arts.

Let's take chiropractic as an example. Because your medical doctor has no training in chiropractic, an opinion on whether you should see a chiropractor is a *personal* opinion. And you should take it as that. A personal opinion would be similar to your neighbor from your cul-de-sac telling their viewpoint or what they have heard about chiropractic. A neighbor may or may not be a good source of information about a healing path.

Some professions that seem to be holistic or bodywork-based are entry paths to The System. Most, but not all, physical therapists, some massage therapists, even some chiropractors can be the funnel to a medical referral that propels you back into the hands of The System. I understand that they are your buddies and want to assist you. And they are. Teaching you new skills, honing your sport performance, or improving your strength, balance, and posture are good things. But if they advise you outside of their expertise, or their usual classroom structure, just nod and smile. If they "should" you, or say there is no possible way the path you are pursuing is valid, or otherwise have too much energy invested in your problem, continue with your class or training and don't ask for explanation. If they want to immediately talk you into a different course of action, be wary. However, if your instructor or trainer says to you merely as an aside, "I did this, and it helped me," with no emotional investment, feel free to investigate.

Have you ever been in the waiting room of a medical office around lunch time and seen an attractive young person carrying a large briefcase? Obviously, this person is not a patient based on the way the staff jokes around with them. They are very friendly with each other. Let me introduce you to the drug representative from a pharmaceutical company, who has come to share samples with the doctor. Conventional medicine and pharmaceutical companies walk hand in hand. It's probably true that medical professionals rarely have time to read the journals that contain drug research, either about new drugs on the market or old drugs with new uses. Sounds reasonable that pharmaceutical companies send out a knowledgeable person with information, right? This is the way that drug information is disseminated. Medications are introduced, or the same old drug gets a reminder to doctors' offices via the friendly briefcase person that brings lunch to the whole staff. Many offices have drug reps of differing companies coordinate with each other, so lunch is provided every day. Every working day of the year. That's right, a free lunch Monday through Friday.

Medical doctors rarely have lunch with an acupuncturist, or homeopath, or nutritional expert to learn what's new. That's not their gig. Pharmaceutical companies are their gig.

Again, there are exceptions. If your medical doctor is one that has one foot in the world of conventional medicine and one foot in the holistic world, they will tell you this without hesitation. If their goal is to see you heal and move away from drugs, you will know it. If you find a medical professional like this, use them as a resource.

Source to Beware #2:
Other People's Opinions

This would include people in your life and the general public. It could be your personal trainer, your kid's athletic trainer at their high school or college, your yoga teacher, your hair stylist, your nail technician, your family, your best friend, or the gal with the twins in the park. A cowboy friend of mine once told me, "Opinions are like elbows. Everybody's got one." People like to show concern, which is nice. But they have a lot of, ya know, elbows. Especially about you. Your father, your mother, your sister, your daughter, your neighbor, your coworkers may feel compelled to share it with you, especially if they don't support your quest. Remember that they haven't done the work that you have.

This is different from a quick, *hey, this helped me,* as I described earlier with my friend Greg. Weird things happen when someone else has an emotional attachment to *your* problem.

Those that are close to you want to help you and do not want to see you suffer. That doesn't mean that their recommendations to you are unadulterated by their own fears and underlying discriminations.

Let's talk about this for a minute. Breaking away from the pack is a scary thing. It is scary for you. And it is scary for those near to you that you are inclined to break away from the pack. This is ancestral reptilian brain behavior. From the dawn of civilization, humans have stayed in groups for safety. Also, shared beliefs and morals, common practices and habits bind us together. When you break away from the group, your friends, your coworkers, your family will see it as an insult to their safety. It's not a rational thought. It's in their DNA. Because of this, they won't know why the feelings of betrayal and rejection of your quest are so strong. It is the most primitive part of our brain that seeks safety from the unknown. And this is okay. It's okay that they don't understand and don't vehemently support the journey. You cannot control it. You cannot control why people say or do what they say and do.

You are making a conscious choice to go out of convention, against the flow of current practices, and that can be scary. But, don't let others' fears become your fear. You are embracing a new way of being and you are allowed to do that. Not only are you allowed to do that, you can be an example to others. Be that example. Let them know that you're still part of their culture, you are still part of their family, you're still part of their group, but there are some things on which you will just have to agree to disagree.

Then there is True Belief. Dr Robert Welch in *Over-diagnosed*,[89] discusses this in relation to early-detection screenings for cancer, osteoporosis, and genetic predispositions, among others. Purportedly these screenings are used to save lives and save money. Many in the healthcare arena deeply believe, to their core, this is the case. Dr. Welch's research proves it may not be true. For our purposes, True Belief refers to those in your life who fight against *your* choices using *their* reasons. They believe that you should 'check with your doctor,' not understanding that medical doctors have no education in chiropractic—or Ayurveda, or a vegan diet, or whatever path you are exploring. These people that are close to you are under the trance of the unrelenting force of The System. This force cannot be conquered by you.

89 Welch, *Over-diagnosed*, 182.

It can only be retreated from. No matter how compelling your own story of healing, no matter the documented studies you invoke, you'll not sway True Belief. The good news is that the True Believer will not sway you either.

For some of you, there are smart and caring people in your life who demand evidence. Holistic health paradigms, by nature of their vitalistic tenants, don't have large RCT studies to prove it. That doesn't mean there is a lack of evidence. *Clinical case studies* are a detailed review of the treatment of individuals, as opposed to large groups of people. These types of articles abound in the journals. Here are just a few titles: "Reduction in Arterial Blood Pressure Following Adjustment of the Atlas to Correct Vertebral Subluxation: A Prospective Longitudinal Cohort Study," (by Torns SR in the *Journal of Upper Cervical Chiropractic Research*, August 11, 2014), or "Resolution of Otitis Media and Nocturnal Enuresis in a 12-Year-Old Patient Following Chiropractic Care to Reduce Vertebral Subluxations: A Case Study and Selected Review of the Literature," (by Marko S. and Marko J. in the *Journal of Pediatric, Maternal & Family Health, Chiropractic*, April 2, 2018.) Although only singular cases, the benefit was clear. The proof was in the pudding, as they say.

Basic science research that proves chiropractic theory is typically published in science journals of various specialized concentrations. An example is this 2014 article published in PLOS One journal, "Definition of the To Be Named Ligament and Vertebrodural Ligament and their Possible Effects on the Circulation of CSF." You can see why this one doesn't make the nightly news. But if you would allow me to explain in kindergarten terms, this *to-be-named ligament* is the reason for the powerful effects of an upper neck spinal adjustment. If a vertebra in your upper neck becomes misaligned, the fluid that surrounds the brain and spinal cord stagnates. This affects the ability of the nerves to fire. If the nerve transmission is disrupted, there is no way that your body can function properly. No way. This research article discussed a possible mechanism to explain how chiropractic works.

The following is a short and incomplete list of journals related to chiropractic research that can be accessed online: *Journal of Vertebral Subluxation (JVSR), Journal of Pediatric, Maternal & Family Health – Chiropractic (JPMFH), Journal of Upper Cervical Chiropractic Research, Annals of Vertebral Subluxation Research, Chiropractic Journal of Australia,* and the *Journal of*

Clinical Chiropractic Pediatrics. If your ultrascience-loving family member is interested, they can obtain a monthly subscription to the *On Purpose* audios. These are succinct and insightful compilations of the relevant journal articles published each month.[90] I've been a subscriber for twenty-plus years.

A Cautionary Tale

That was $1,000 of homeopathic remedies she poured down the drain, I thought. *And she's still sick.* The reason? Her mother doesn't understand homeopathy. Trudie does. She understands that the homeopathic remedies recommended to her contain a minuscule amount of toxic substance to compel your body to wage war. In her case the war is against a nasty antibiotic-resistant germ she contracted while having emergency surgery six months prior. She had fallen off a roof while volunteering in Southeast Asia and cracked her cheekbone. Trudie understands, at least theoretically, how homeopathic remedies work. She had done her term paper on it for her AP biology class as a senior. Her mom, a hospital administrator, is a True Believer in conventional medicine. Trudie knows that she can't change her mom, and she has chosen to keep the peace at home by continuing on the conventional medicine path. They, the doctors, say she is close to healed. Unfortunately, she is acutely aware that she is not, based on the symptoms of fatigue, digestive upset, and joint pain still plaguing her. That's a tough conundrum to manage at nineteen years old.

This is a tough one at any age, actually. Your ability to remain on task, to remain true to the mission, will be tested. Respect for others' beliefs is important, but it is imperative that others respect your desire to search both inside and outside of the conventional medical system. Be kind, but remember Mission You is paramount.

As you and I travel this journey together, I have to ask: My friend, how are you doing? You may be running into brick-wall situations like Trudie. Food choices may be a challenge to you right now, as if bad stuff lurks in all the things that are *supposed* to be good for you. You may be experienc-

---

90 On Purpose, LLC, 3740 Boiling Springs Hwy #108, Boiling Springs SC 29316. www.chiroonpurpose.com.

ing detox symptoms of tiredness and crabbiness. The list of supplements you prep each day may suddenly seem ridiculous. No matter what form of cruddy-ness you are going through, please, take a moment. Breathe in and out slowly and deeply. And again, in and out. Let's remember the life you are fighting for. Find the list of key motivators you created in Chapter 1. Look inside the bathroom cabinet for that note and re-stick it to the mirror. Where is that recording you made? Make a point to listen. Were you the one that created the vision board? Hang it prominently. I know it's hard. Healing has become your hobby—which is kind of a drag. But your life awaits. Hang in there.

Remember the list you've been compiling of resources? The people who are propelling you along your journey? They have been where you are, right now. Reach out to them and discuss your stumbling blocks. I would pinky-bet they can offer some guidance.

Don't assume that others have not seen the changes you've made thus far. Ask for feedback from those that support you. The most compelling evidence of a successful mission is the outward changes, the changes others see. Even True Believers may bend a little bit.

Source to Beware #3:
Advertising, the Media, and (Surprisingly) Research

"Honey ... how many people do you know who are blind?" I asked my husband, who was in the kitchen having just picked up the dinner dishes. I was in the TV room with the dog.

"Uhhh ... none ... I think.... Why?"

"I know one. Well, two if you count my Uncle Shorty who died twenty-five years ago. The reason I ask is there's been this commercial on TV for the last two months for a new drug for Non-24 Syndrome. Is there really so many blind people that this drug deserves to be advertised every night?"

My pondering that night was answered about six months later when I read Elizabeth Rosenthal's book, *An American Sickness: How Healthcare Became Big Business and How you Can Take it Back.* In Chapter 4, "The

Age of Pharmaceuticals," subchapter: "Non-24, it pays to Advertise," she discusses the small population of Americans who are completely blind, and because they cannot see sunlight, lose the normal rhythm of sleepiness and wakefulness. Certainly, it is a debilitating disease.

In 2014, a drug was released to market that targeted Non-24 and the small number of people who suffered with it. The drug influences receptors for melatonin, a hormone which is produced by the pineal gland in the brain. Melatonin, the hormone which partly governs our sleep/wake cycle is thought to be regulated by the sunlight. If someone is completely blind, they may lose the influence that light has on them. For many people, even those with Non-24, taking a supplemental capsule of melatonin forty-five minutes prior to bedtime can be beneficial. Since it occurs in nature, it is not a patentable product.

The FDA approval process requires that drug companies prove the drug is safe, and that it works better than placebo (a sugar pill). The drugs do *not* need to be proven to work better than other drugs available, or naturally occurring products. In this case the naturally occurring product is melatonin. It works similarly to the drug, only better.

Interestingly, the rules, as written, *forced* FDA advisers to approve the drug for release despite knowing that melatonin could be a better choice. It's also cheaper. Once the drug was approved to market, the price was set to $8,000 for a month's supply, or $267.00 per pill. Melatonin can be bought at a local drug store chain for $1.50 per month, or five cents a pill.

Once a medication is approved, prescriptions can be written off-label, meaning doctors can recommend it for any symptom. In the Non-24 case, this drug can be prescribed for any sleep disorder, including jet lag.[91] Jet leg even has a fancy Latin diagnosis: desynchronosis. (Test your Latin word origin search skills on that one.) A quick internet query of jet lag led me to an article. It appeared on the first page of internet searches where The System lives. It had some good info in spite of that. Buried within it is a mention of melatonin. But, according to the article, melatonin is said to lack research to verify its effectiveness. Hmmm, interesting. The next sentence

---

91   Rosenthal, *An American Sickness*, 101.

said that drug therapies "may be available." I suppose you would have to "ask your doctor" for the $267.00-per-pill prescription.

What should be advertised, at least on every flight overseas is our course called Jet Lag No More.[92] It's true, jet lag can be completely eliminated by using acupressure points. And once you buy the program and learn it, it's free. Free for future travel, your family, your travel buds, and the guy sitting next to you in seat 24B. It doesn't cost $1.50 a month, and certainly not $8,000.

It is possible that melatonin is a better choice, at a lower price (by thousands.) Yet with no commercial to tell you, how would you know? The advertising you see every day is designed to sell you something, not teach you something. We are inundated with ads made to look like education. It is not. That's our responsibility. We must explore and learn things ourselves.

Drug ads on the network and cable news channels are beautifully done, with compelling stories, like the Non-24 commercial. And those work. The medication for Non-24 was expected to bring in $140 million in 2019 alone, with sales climbing. That's not as huge as the heavy hitter, cholesterol-lowering statin drugs which have been leading the pack for years. I'm thinking that the advertising industry must love the pharmaceutical industry. They get to showcase their most creative minds. The pharmaceutical companies are clients that always return with work to be done and lots of money to spend. The ad makers don't care if a five-cent melatonin pill works better. They are most concerned with their bottom line: paying the bills and satisfying their stockholders. They are part of The System. Good, better, cheaper alternatives don't get to buy expensive advertising. These are not the darlings bringing home the bacon. The moral question about what is better for the public, or what is better for you, the individual, is not even asked. You and your Stealth Health quest are not part of the equation. Naturally occurring products cannot be patented. No singular company can make a bajillion dollars from it, as in the case of melatonin. So therefore, no big advertising campaigns are launched. The only thing you will absorb from any advertisement is what they *want* you to believe. It's not the whole truth.

TV and cable stations generate income from selling advertising spots.

---

92 www.drnancytrimboli.com

Companies that buy time during television shows pay between $150,000 to nearly $700,000 for a single airing. Each thirty-second commercial pays for the news anchors, the film crew, the producers, the behind-the-scenes staff, the building where they film, the news vans sent out on location, and all the rest. And let's not forget the stockholders and other investors. The financial benefit is so great that to expose the charade of a drug being outperformed by a supplement would be self-destructive. If the news shows were to have lengthy discussions about the loopholes in FDA regulations that don't require new meds to be any better than the existing, or to be compared to other remedies prior to being released to market, it would probably need to lay off all of their news anchors and support staff. The fact that they stay quiet about the truth that melatonin is just as good as the Non-24 medication keeps everyone employed. If your favorite news anchor were to say during her nightly sign off, "Oh, and remember the mistruth of high cholesterol being linked to heart disease is based on a poorly charted graph from the 1920s.[93] Statin drugs might be creating more disease than it's preventing. But we're not quite sure because no one will pay for that research. Good night and sleep tight! We'll be back for our evening broadcast tomorrow."

Pharmaceutical companies make a product. The advertising industry creates the ads that sell that product. The news programs benefit from the sale of that advertising time. Your well-being does not come into play. When people are sick, money is put into the cycle, and the The System becomes stronger.

Being a business owner, I like to say that people vote with their feet. No focus groups or online surveys will predict how people will act in any situation. If all choices were equally available and there were no financial obstacles (no advertising for either side), what would you imagine the outcome to be if we stacked holistic care against drug-based conventional medical care? It may never happen, but I would love to see the results of *that* study.

---

93 *Statin Nation*, directed by Justin Smith. (2012)

Research that is really advertising

For every research headline that supports a concept, there is another that will conclude the opposite. Or, it seems that way. Eat unripe bananas. Eat boiled bananas. Take vitamin D. Vitamin D is toxic. Vitamin D is not a vitamin. You can't win.

How do you navigate research studies that make headlines? For one, you may need to ignore those. Research studies on nutritional supplements can go awry for a variety of reasons. The supplement may have been given at the wrong time, to the wrong people, in the wrong dose, or in the wrong form. In the case of a CoQ10 supplement study, cardiac patients were given a nonabsorbable form of the vitamin. The conclusion of the study was that CoQ10 did not work.[94] In two research studies, participants were given the supplement echinacea at the wrong time. It was given to patients who had already succumbed to the illness.[95] Echinacea works best given prior to the start of cold or flu symptoms. Because natural remedies are specific for each person, and do not treat a diagnosis, researching a holistic treatment on a thousand people with the same diagnosis may not prove anything. Research studies are set up to use the conventional medical model and are aimed at proving or disproving treatments for a diagnosis. The two do not mix.

All the conflicting information paralyzes us, shatters our trust in any information and funnels us back into The System. Headlines catch our attention and distract us from the real issues. Drama, controversy, and fear sell advertising. That's why we listen, watch, or read the news. It's as if we don't have enough drama in our lives already.

Often studies receive media time on internet news sites, headlines, and the nightly news that prove such things as a 50% drop in your risk of such-and-such, or an 11% improvement in so-and-so. And I bet it caught your attention. Unless you go to the actual journal article quoted, you can't be sure of its significance. A 50% drop in risk could be a difference between

---

94 Sinatra, Stephen, *Sinatra Solution: Metabolic Cardiology* (California: Basic Health Publishing, 2008), audio version.

95 National Center for Complementary and Integrative Health. U.S. Department of Health & Human Services. National Institutes of Health. USA.gov. *Three Studies Find Echinacea Ineffective Against the Common Cold*, 2005. Last modified January 27, 2015. Accessed August 23, 2019. https://nccih.nih.gov/research/results/spotlight/051805.htm.

.002% (two one-thousandths of a percent) of the population getting a snake bite when going for a hike versus .001% if they stopped for a fudge sundae on the way. It's not statistically significant. The fact is that over 99% of us hikers will never be bitten by a snake.

The only statistics you should regard are those that report a change of double or more. Certainly a change of ten-times is a major heads-up. Ignore all the studies that want to scare you or lead you to action by reporting a double-digit *percentage* increase or decrease. These studies may have gotten the researchers a published paper, but the causal relationship between the two things, whether it is Vitamin E and cardiac health, or coffee and cancer prevention, is not proven. Dr. Robert Welch in *Less Medicine, More Health*, describes the Hill criteria, which helps to determine if one event created another event.[96] I'll spare you the lesson in statistics. Graduations of causality exist from weak association to strong association like a sliding scale. A risk or benefit less than two-fold indicate a weak association. If it's a weak association, you can go back to eating your broccoli, which is 1000% better than a hundred-calorie snack bag of anything.

In today's world, as much as it breaks my heart to say, scientific literature can be swayed. Not all of it is swayed, and not even most of it, yet it never should be susceptible to even the slightest insinuation. Jim Oschman, PhD and researcher, is the author of *Energy Medicine: The Scientific Basis*. In a January 2019 interview with Dr. Christopher Kent and Dr. Patrick Gentempo on the *On Purpose* monthly audio series, he states, "I've been saddened by the way science has been misused. We have … damaged the integrity of science when … medical doctors … put their names on papers, published in support of using a particular drug. They have not done any of the research. They have sold their name and their prestige … That is not acceptable … Science is meant to find out what is going on … to have no value judgement or vested interest. Vested interests have taken over science… That's a tragedy." Dr. Oschman is referring to the practice of "ghostwriting."[97] Authors hired by pharmaceutical companies write the arti-

---

96 Welch, Gilbert *Less Medicine, More Health*. (Massachusetts: Beacon Press, 2015), 11.

97 Sismondo, Sergio, "Ghost Management: How Much of the Medical Literature is Shaped Behind the Scenes by the Pharmaceutical Industry?" *PloS Medicine* 4(9) (2007): e286. Accessed August 3, 2019. doi: 10.1371/journal.pmed.0040286.

cles but make it appear that an influential medical doctor or academic did the research. In exchange, the medical doctors are compensated. Although a small portion of all journal submissions, it is a disturbing trend that must infuriate those people who have dedicated their life to making a difference and struggle to find funding.

Who pays to keep the lights on?

There is economics involved in publishing research, and it must be paid by someone. Just like any business or household, there's bills to pay: payroll for the scientists, mathematicians, chemists, lab assistants, and janitors, the rent of the physical space in which they work, the electricity, the waste disposal, and the computers. It's expensive. Approval for research grant money is bestowed by the True Believers that set up The System. Most grant writers who seek research money follow the same path of those before them in the hopes of keeping their labs going.[98] This does not allow for those with contradictory ideas to get much attention. Even if a grant is awarded one time in an effort to explore a holistic avenue and shows positive results, obtaining money for follow up studies is unlikely.

This is probably the reason you rarely hear about big research projects studying the efficiency and cost savings with using chiropractic. The research on how homeopathy may help people with cancer and Lyme disease cannot be found. The investigations into the effectiveness of holistic remedies is sparse. And if by chance a small study is published, the required follow-up study won't happen. The reason: nobody's paying for it. Because researching nonpatentable, natural remedies doesn't feed the cycle of The System.

The System relies on us to be either sick or afraid of becoming sick. Not all, but much of research promulgated by the media, either by default or by design, supports testing centers, treatment centers, pharmaceutical companies, device makers of all types, academia and schools, career centers of the medical support personnel, even computer software and hardware creators, manufacturers, and maintenance. Elizabeth Rosenthal, in *An American Sick-*

---

98   Welch, *Over-diagnosed*, 158.

ness, discusses the infiltration of for-profit venture capitalists into projects funded by JDRF (previously the Juvenile Diabetes Research Foundation) and the Cystic Fibrosis Foundation.[99] I'm not sure what the solution is. But I do know one thing. Making profits from the prolongation of disease and infirmity removes the desire to cure it. And people who become healthy outside of The System do not feed the conglomerate, venture-capitalist loving, money-making machine. Natural remedies that use your body's inborn ability to heal run counter to it.

Having been college roommates and friends with those on the firing lines of research, I know the tireless warriors working in the labs are not the ones to blame. They are the ones to be applauded for the efforts to find answers. These are brilliant minds who love the view through the lens of a microscope more than a sunset, who can banter about "cotransport by symporters and antiporters" over morning coffee (I could not), who would fight to the death for the privilege to investigate a hypothesis of the neurophysiology of Fragile X Syndrome (that's out of my league as well), or a collaboration on movement disorders apparent in neurodegenerative diseases. (The last two are projects a former employee, now PhD candidate, is working on.) Their overarching theme is the improvement of human life. They are part of the solution. As the next generation comes up through the ranks of these labs, their childhood and adolescent experiences of their chiropractic adjustments may open the vistas to further explore ways to use safe, effective, holistic treatments. I have confidence they will.

Mission You: Take Action

- Consider the following:

    - Has a trusted person made suggestions that seem foreign? Would you consider investigating that option?

    - Are you being swayed by someone, a friend, coworker, family member, who has their own agenda for you? Is your intuition telling you, even warning you about their interference? Or

---

99 Rosenthal, *An American Sickness*, 183-190.

is their interaction helpful and illustrating positive steps you can take?

- Are you running in circles because you have too many people contributing ideas?

- Remember to use the *My Healthcare Arsenal* workbook page from www.DrNancyTrimboli.com to organize your resources. Refer to this list repeatedly. As Mission You evolves, your needs will change. And, those around you struggling to solve *their* mysteries will begin to ask for *your* secrets. Become their ally and share your arsenal. Go to our *Trimboli Insiders Group* on Facebook to share your resources, the members of your healthcare arsenal, and your triumphs.

Chapter 7

TWELVE WAYS TO ESCAPE
THE HOLD OF THE SYSTEM

ONCE YOU HAVE seen The System for what it is, there is no turning back, no ability to turn off that awareness. You are emboldened with your new powerful questions: **What if I Could Heal?, Why?,** and **Where are my Resources?** Those questions will bring you profound answers as you move along the path.

You'll learn that you are not alone. Using your resources will become second nature. Others are all around you on parallel journeys. They come into plain view once you are free of The System. Because both of you have made the commitment, there is instant comradery and information to share. This is the most satisfying part of being the hero of this spy story. The thriller, heart-pounding scenes are over. You have made the transition to unravel the mystery of you. Revel in the joy of it.

Yet this story is not over. Your challenges with health are not behind you. The System is still all around. You may falter, or The System may trick you back into its clutches. But alliances with like-minded people will grow as your knowledge grows. The resources you have used in the past will continue to remain resources and will help you choose better options. Plus, the knowledge of those people grows over time as they learn, and they will share that with you. Nothing is stagnant. Your need to pull away from The System grows stronger each day as you expand your thinking, your circle of influence, and strive to make better choices.

Jason Bourne may never uncover the reasons that he was targeted for extinction. Even those remotely associated with him were in the crosshairs of his enemies. In the same way, we as Americans fall prey to products, specifically foods with ingredients that are designed to addict us without our health in mind. Our families are subjected to the same perturbed way of life.

Sugar is the most obvious chemical food additive that causes us to become sicker and diminish our wellbeing. Sugar is proven to be linked to diabetes, altered immune responses, including inflammation, depression, heart disease, dementia, and shorter life expectancy.[100,101,102] Yet, behind the facade of protecting public welfare, the FDA allows processed foods to be rife with sugar. Even children are set up for a life of infirmity by being the target audience for ads selling breakfast foods that have more sugar per ounce than soft drinks.[103]

Other hidden additives threaten to destroy our sense of self and happiness. One of these is flavor enhancers which are neurotoxins[104] and can create anxiety, depression, irritability, worry, and violent behavior. One serving of these flavor enhancers can create a craving for it. Each snack chip you eat turns your brain into an addict. You can break free by refusing to ingest the poison. At first it may be difficult because you are addicted. By saying no, and leaving behind the addiction, you say yes to temporary withdrawal symptoms that may be uncomfortable. But you are prepared. You are willing to endure that sacrifice. Just like 007 in all the reincarnations of James Bond, you never back down from your fight. James Bond never says no. Old, bad habits of yours will try to force you back into The System. New habits will propel you away from the hold of The System. Bigger things are at stake here. The snack chip will have to stay in the bag.

100 *Murray, Encyclopedia of Natural Medicine,* 174

101 Murray, Michael, *What the Drug Companies Won't Tell You and Your Doctor Doesn't Know* (New York: Atria Paperbacks, a Division of Simon & Schuster, 2009), 163.

102 Perlmutter, David, *Grain Brain: The Surprising Truth about Wheat, Carbs, and Sugar—Your Brain's Silent Killers* (New York: Little, Brown Spark, 2013)

103 Emond, Jennifer, et al. "Exposure to Child-Directed TV Advertising and Preschoolers' Intake of Advertised Cereals," *American Journal of Preventative Medicine* 56 no.2 (2019): e35-e43, accessed August 25, 2019, doi: https://doi.org/10.1016/j.amepre.2018.09.015.

104 Simontacchi, *Crazy Makers,* 102-106.

Emerging Victorious

All good things take time. You have taken risks in your journey; you have put yourself in peril at times. Some previous friends may no longer be in your inner circle because as you evolve, you leave others behind. Perhaps you have created a whole new world of friends and life influencers. You may have *become* an influencer. Seeing a better way toward healing and health has given you an updated perspective and changed your mindset about how that can be achieved.

You can see The System and its many players as something to avoid. The prevailing "wisdom" is now full of holes. The news, whether read or heard or watched, abounds with mistruths that push you to less healthy choices. Advertisers are amazing talents in the way they can tap into our human fears and worldly wants. Look upon their work, the advertisements in their various forms, as something to behold with the fascination of a scientific observation. The advertisers want you to believe their product is the best, or the *only* option. You and I both know better.

Perhaps you are re-evaluating what products you are using on your skin, your hair, and in your home. Can you find something less toxic, better for you, and better for the family? Medical recommendations and approaches are now seen as just one choice in a myriad of choices, and you evaluate it for its benefits and risks. The health book that your friend recommended is infinitely more helpful than the medical appointment for which you waited six months. Just like Jason Bourne, by avoiding The System, you can live your life freely in the sunshine, with your favorite girl, on a beach renting scooters to tourists.

#1 Carve Out the Time

It may be an application on your phone, it may be the paper kind on the wall, or the white board you keep for the family. Taking care of yourself takes time. Some of your weekly or monthly habits do not serve you. Removing items from your calendar will free up space to complete Mission You. Say "no" to some things so you can say "yes" to Mission You. You'll need stolen moments to research and read. Leave available time slots to see new health professionals. Recruit the kids to help implement strategies. Make lists to arrange your grocery shopping as it will be different than the past. Alert the family to show reverence for your sleep time. At all times the primary focus is Mission You.

When you become aware of The System all around you, your choices in entertainment will naturally alter. You will see the way The System infiltrates your favorite shows and movies. The advertising in your search engines will repulse you. Honor that awareness. Avoid those shows and movies. Change your ad choices in your search engine. Remove that advertising from your vision.

#2 Choose Positivity

We are strongly influenced by those that surround us on a daily basis. Be sure that they honor your soul, add to your enthusiasm, and stimulate you mentally. Resolve to input good things into your psyche and mind. If painting makes your day better, do that. If a tai chi class every Saturday soothes you and makes you a better person, do that. Does having lunch with specific friends once a month keep you focused on your goals when everything else in life goes awry? Put that in your calendar as a non-negotiable appointment.

Stay away from fear. Stay away from drama. Stay away from negativity. Nothing good comes of it. If you have teenagers, do the best you can. They grow up and become good people. Hang in there.

At times we are unsure of how people affect us. After spending time with someone, ask yourself: Does this person cause me to feel creative and challenge me to think bigger, or do conversations with this person cause me to feel worried, self-conscious, judged, or judgmental? If it is the latter, this is not a relationship that fuels your journey. You have my permission to cut ties or, at least, to limit time with that person.

#3 Excuse Me, Your Vitality is Showing

As you have moved along in Mission You to unravel the mystery of you, your health and energy have improved. This shows on your face. Others can see it. They want what you have. The System insists that we all feel broken down, tired, and unresourceful. If we are too tired and distracted to seek a better way, we succumb to our old ways. When others see your energy strengthen and vitality bloom, they crave that. Share with them what you have learned. Be one of those people who says, "I did this. It really helped me. You might want to try it." As we align with like-minded people traveling on parallel paths to wellness, the Stealth Health movement will strengthen, and the quicker The System will topple.

As you investigate and experience the vitalistic avenues of healing, you will hear the term "wellness care" and begin to understand the concepts of strengthening the body to prevent disease. As one of my associate chiropractors once said to me, "If Americans would get bodywork done on a regular basis, seventy-five percent of the health problems in the U.S. would disappear." Can research support this hypothesis? Not specifically, because you can't prove what doesn't happen, meaning what's been prevented. Bodywork such as chiropractic care, massage, and other hands-on approaches are simple things that can have huge ramifications.

Author of *Energy Medicine: The Scientific Basis*, Dr. Jim Oschman, agrees. In a recorded conversation, he stated, "A massage every week is a great thing to do. I go to my acupuncturist, when I feel good, for a tune-up…. I go see my chiropractor when I feel fine. This makes sense to me…. our healthcare system needs to recognize the total value of this. People who follow this strategy are going to be the ones who are healthy, happy, … and who are going to live the lives they want … to a ripe old age."[105]

Conventional medical approaches work by addressing a symptom, the disease, and the diagnosis. The holistic paradigm takes a different approach. Healing comes from within by improving overall function and tapping into the body's natural regenerative ability. Almost always, opportunities exist to make improvements. Toxins abound in our water, food, and air.

---

105 Jim Oschman, "Philosophy," *On Purpose* monthly audio recording with Christopher Kent, DC and Patrick Gentempo, DC (January 2019)

Emotional stresses are a way of life and are constant. Structurally, our environment is horrible. Our chairs are better suited for a bag of groceries than our behinds. Our cars force us into a poor sedentary posture. Then layer on the emotional stress of driving. Family dynamics have changed so that, frequently, three generations live in one home. Helping with your elderly parent or your grandchild takes an emotional and physical toll. Without the kids down the block offering help with leaves and snow removal in exchange for spending money, maintenance of our homes and yards disrupts not only our moods but our body's alignment too. Exercise and playing sports is great for the mind and the body, but it is opportunity for the occasional minor, or major, injury.

Letting these structural, energy, neural, and other interferences remain will create symptoms and problems. Undoing these destructive forces puts us closer to an optimal state. Holistic health providers detect and correct these underlying, nonsymptomatic distortions. Going through life holding onto the imbalances and interferences is asking for trouble. It is like a ticking time bomb. Symptoms and problems will result if left uncorrected. It's not a matter of if, but when. For some, it becomes a race against time to find the bomb and clip the correct wires to regain health. For others, the existence of the bomb is ignored or contested, and it explodes.

Our Mission You hero does not do that. You are the hero that knows the bomb exists and that it is up to you to disarm it. You trust your intel. You understand cause and effect. An action leads to an outcome. Your life, full of stresses, creates chaos in your body. To achieve a greater state of wellbeing, clearing the interferences is essential. Body work will reward you beyond what any words can muster. Just do it.

A New Optimum

Alanna was happily talking with me about her success with chiropractic for not only her original complaint of neck pain, but also the other side benefits she was experiencing.

"I always blamed the M.S. for my leg pain at night and the way my leg swings when I walk. I always assumed my left leg was shorter because of the pin in my hip from my old injury. And, the kicker is, I use alternative medicine. My functional doctor, who is also a neurologist, has taught me to control my symptoms with diet and exercise. I couldn't tolerate the M.S. medications; they tore me up. But even knowing all of that and teaching my support group how to use alternative methods, I didn't realize I needed chiropractic care. I had no idea that chiropractic could do so much. I've had ten adjustments so far and I walked three-quarters of a mile at the lake this weekend, up and down hills, and I haven't done that for twenty years! This has been a miracle."

#4 Yup, You Guessed It, Use Chiropractic

Find yourself a true chiropractor who will assess your spine and nerve system to remove interferences in nerve transmission. For those of you who may not know what chiropractic is, I'll explain. Just for fun try this explanation on a four-year-old. I'm not insulting your intelligence. Kids innately understand the basic concept. Adults want it to be complicated. Rest assured that the science, philosophy, and art of chiropractic is complex and deserves the rigorous five-year academic program of the doctorate degree. But the basic concepts are straight-forward. Are you ready with your favorite four-year-old?

Your body has electrical power in it to make everything work. It has power because you are different than a rock or a chair or a table; you have life. (Ask them if they know this. They do.) All the power comes from the brain. (This is where you'll lose most four-year-olds, unless you give them a hint, such as pointing to your head.) The power travels from your brain to your body by going through a network of wires that's inside your spine that come out from between each bone in your back. These wires are called nerves. (This is not a required fact in the four-year-old world.) Each bump on your back is a separate bone. (This one is always new information.) What do you think would happen if one of these little bones shifted out of place just enough to *stop* the electrical power from getting through? (With my hands in a prayer position, I rotate my palms opposite ways then clap. *Clap!*) Do you think that's a good thing? Or a bad thing? That's right, it's a bad thing. (All four-year-olds know it's a bad thing when the power is stopped.) No matter where that nerve goes in your body, whether it's your tummy, or your nose, or your toes, that part can't work correctly if the power is not getting through. My job as a chiropractor is to fix your back so all your power can work. (Most kids at this point cannot wait for me to check their power.)

The System has targeted chiropractic for elimination nearly since its inception. This is because chiropractic works. The best part about chiropractic is the side *benefits*. Drugs have side effects, detrimental side effects. Chiropractic has side benefits. As an example, you may consult with a chiropractor for lower back pain and find that as the nerves of the lower back are cleared, your digestion and elimination improve.[106] The nerves of the lower back go to everything from your waist to the floor. As those nerves are cleared with the adjustments, the pain improves, and clearing those nerves allows all functions of those nerves to improve as well. Chiropractic adjustments are a simple action to take, yet the effects are profound.

There are dozens of ways chiropractors analyze and restore nerve transmission and improve spinal alignment. Adjustment styles range from extremely light touch to the high velocity, low amplitude manipulations typically associated with chiropractic. On the light touch end of the spectrum there is nearly zero force, as in the amount of pressure you would use to touch a baby's nose. On the opposite end of the spectrum there is enough force to cause a popping noise in the vertebral joints. All the chiropractic adjustment techniques work. The technique that works best for you is a combination of what's appropriate for your body plus your preference. To assist you in this process, go to my YouTube channel for this video: "How to Find the Best Chiropractor for You."[107]

Find an adjustment style that you like. If the chiropractor has answers for your three powerful questions (**What if I Could Heal?, Why?,** and **Where are my Resources?**) and propels you on your steps to solve Mission

106 Angus, Katherine, Sepideh Asghaifar, and Brian Gleberzon, "What effect does chiropractic treatment have on gastrointestinal (GI) disorders: a narrative review of the literature," *The Journal of the Canadian Chiropractic Association* 59 no.2 (2015):122-133, accessed August 25, 2019. https://www.ncbi.nlm.nih.gov/pmc/articles/PMC4486990.

107 Trimboli, Nancy "How to Choose the Best Chiropractor for You." *YouTube*. Video File. October 1, 2018. https://www.youtube.com/watch?v=gZrqDGJ8v7U.

You, follow through with the care plan that they suggest. Stay on maintenance chiropractic care thereafter.

#5 Massage, Not Just for Spas

Massage therapy, especially when used routinely, can have an increasing benefit for the body by relaxing spasm and improving the mobility of the joints. You'll be able to move better during your average day. Relaxation or spa-like massage can reduce stress and improve blood flow to muscles and clear toxins. Therapeutic massage is targeted to certain muscle groups for repetitive-use muscle strain, new injury, or chronic pain from previous injury. Specialized techniques such as lymphatic drainage, CranioSacral therapy, and Myofascial Release are helpful for other health challenges and general wellness. Plan on a monthly massage to keep healthy.

#6 Body Humors, Currents, and Frequencies

Ancient healing arts, those that have been known to be in use for thousands of years, attempt to balance our nonphysical vital forces to promote health. Ayurveda examines the doshas. Energy medicine opens chakras. Acupuncture is a component of traditional Chinese medicine and strives to restore the flow of chi through twenty meridians. All of these systems, and many others, are vitalistic in philosophy. These are foreign to most of us having been raised in The System, a mechanistic society strongly influenced by the Industrial Age of automobiles and manufacturing. The concepts run counter to the algorithms of a conventional medical practitioner, unless they have committed themselves to study vitalistic methods. As I compile interviews with practitioners inside these healing arts, you'll have access to firsthand information. Check my website for details on how this will become available to you. If you decide to research vitalistic healing philosophies online, skip immediately to page four of the results. The conjecture on pages one through three are a fine example of The System at work. That alone should tell you how powerful this work must be.

I understand your uncomfortableness with these topics. As a chiropractor, I work with my hands, and also my observational skills. I can see imbalances in the structure of someone and feel the differences in muscle and skin of the affected regions. The fields of energy are such that, although I can't explain it or see it, I know it's there. We're friends here, so let's just say it, it's weird. It may seem a little hokey. Energy work and other ancient healing arts may not be the right path for you. That's okay. If, however, your quest to wellness repeatedly diverts you to a practitioner of a type of energy medicine, allow yourself at least a cursory investigation. An answer may be waiting to be discovered, or this new member of your healthcare arsenal can perhaps illuminate a worthwhile path.

#7 Be *That Guy* that Eats Only Broccoli at Work

Eat right for you. You may be a type that thrives on meat. Or, you may do well with a vegan way of eating. Your biochemistry is unique to you and is based on your history and your genealogy. You are a product of your ancestors. Regardless of what you choose, once you know yourself, stick with the plan.

No one does well with a diet full of sugar (even hidden sugar) or food additives. No one should be eating food from a package on a regular basis. This includes drinks, powders, bars, and other whatnot that are purportedly natural, organic, vegan, keto, or whatever catchphrase attracts you. My rule is to read the label—the ingredients. If there is something on the label I cannot pronounce, or would not be found in a normal kitchen, I leave it on the shelf. Exceptions may be amino acid powders, but still I am very picky.

Eating clean means that the easiest, fastest route to a meal rarely exists unless you plan ahead. Stock your refrigerator, freezer, and pantry with healthy basics. Shop frequently. Whole foods that closely resemble how it existed in nature is my definition of a clean diet. A snack is a handful of nuts—raw or roasted with no additional seasoning other than sea salt. A salad is sometimes a pile of fresh green beans or kale massaged with olive oil and sprinkled with herbs. It will take time to prepare. It's not cheap. It's not convenient. But, neither is the medical treatment you'll need if you don't eat right. As you notice your symptoms recede and your energy improve, you will not only find the motivation to do it, you'll feel cheated when you don't.

Get an IG-g food allergy test done to determine if you are sensitive to any foods or additives. These types of food sensitivities have a delayed reaction by up to four days and can have a sneaky bad effect on your health. It could be a food that you eat regularly and, ironically, may be a food that you are attracted to. Even good foods can produce a response. Garlic, citrus fruits, and kidney beans are some that I've seen show up on these tests. Once eradicated, stubborn symptoms subside.

While on Mission You and fixing yourself, nutritional supplements can be complex. Take the time to understand the supplements you are taking. Use muscle testing[108] to know what is right for you, right now, in this moment. Regaining health can require that you feed yourself differently. It may mean that you are on fistfuls of supplements for a time. But once Mission You is complete, a simple personalized daily supplement regimen can keep you healthy and happy.

#8 Count Your Ounces, then Drink Them

Your daily intake of water should equal half your body weight in ounces. If you weigh 160 pounds, your daily water requirement is 80 ounces. Get accustomed to room temperature water in 16-ounce servings. You can then drink a lot and quickly with no brain freeze. Drink two cups at a time and you only need to remember to drink water five times a day: upon waking, before lunch, midafternoon, before dinner, and before bed. If you are drinking extra ounces of water due to your weight, add midmorning, early afternoon, and early evening water portions. Intake of caffeine or alcohol will need to be replaced by water. If you have a 12-ounce cup of coffee, add 12 ounces of water to your daily requirement. Paradoxically, when imbibing the proper amount, you will notice thirst throughout the day, and even at night. Add a squeeze of lemon in your water to help the

---

108 Eden, Donna, Energy Medicine (New York: Tarcher / Putnam a member of Penguin Putnam, 1999), pp. 44-59.

acid-alkaline balance of your body and help to curb those nasty sugar and carbohydrate withdrawal cravings. Reverse osmosis is the best water to drink as it removes bacteria and heavy metals but leaves the minerals behind for your body to utilize. Metal or glass containers are optimal. Try your best to not store your water in plastic.

#9 The Activity of Sleep

We are as a society, dictated by our to-do lists. What if, in sleep, we checked more boxes than in our awake time? Dr. Matthew Walker, in his book, *Why We Sleep,* describes the amazing effects that sleep can have on our creativity, emotional state, learning and retention, organ function and repair, and happiness.[109] All living creatures partake in some form of sleep to regenerate. Here are some simple sleep rules. Adhere to nearly the same bedtime and wake time each day. Paradoxically, going outside in the morning will help you sleep at night. It improves the cortisol/melatonin hormone balance to allow greater attentiveness during the day and sleepiness at night. Avoid blue light screens two hours before bed. Keep your room cool and close out all light. Take a warm shower, bath, or hot tub dip prior to bed. Use essential oils for relaxation. Prepare for bedtime with a change of clothes into your pajamas, use your bedroom for only sleeping (not for work or to read or to watch TV), and soften the lights. Include meditation, prayer, or voicing gratitude as part of your daily routine to rest your mind, let go of worry, and reduce stress.[110]

---

109 Walker, Matthew, *Why We Sleep: Unlocking the Power of Sleep and Dreams* (New York: Scribner, and imprint of Simon & Schuster, 2017)

110 Trimboli, Nancy. "Ten Things to do Before 10 p.m.," *YouTube*. January 19, 2019. https://www.youtube.com/watch?v=NJA88Sjpvss&t=157s.

#10 Do Something, *Anything*!

We are all busy yet spend excessive amounts of time sitting at our desks and while driving. It has deleterious effects on our psyche and our health. Use movement to counteract this. You may be one that loves exercise. Great, you have this covered. If you do not, don't fret. Just do something, really anything. It could be a walk around your yard or through the neighborhood early in the morning. Go out and pull weeds, take a friend's dog for a walk, or help in a soup kitchen. Find your activity. Look through the local parks department newsletter for introductory classes into dance, swimming, pickleball, tae kwon do, yoga. Do something that makes you happy. Do something that not only moves air in and out of your lungs but also removes the stale air from the base of your lungs. Use your muscles. And even if you do a job that is physical, you need to move your body to work and challenge your muscles in a different way. Release stress and improve your balance through exercise. Sweat a little to release toxins and for emotional release.

#11 Get the Sludge Out

No matter where you turn, there are toxins. Our bodies are meant to handle some toxins, but, in our world today, we are overloaded. Many we can control, most we cannot. Agriculture, commerce, industry, and transportation put chemicals into our environment that are unavoidable. Do what you can in your immediate space to minimize toxin exposure. Care about the chemicals you put on your skin. Petroleum byproducts used in cosmetics and lotions are forbidden in other countries. Seek out products that do not use petrolatum or petroleum. Nontoxic household cleaning products can replace most, if not all, the current toxic ones you use. Outdoor chemicals for weed and pest control can be traded for cheaper, friendlier alternatives. Research and replace.

When you are intent on a healing process, you must give your body the opportunity to shed all the damaged tissue. Also, as we heal, our body recognizes that the gunk it has been holding onto needs to go. Our liver, our lungs, and our skin excrete those toxins, so caring for those organs will aid in cleansing. Use supplements for your liver or do deep yogic breathing with assistance from an expert. Sweating helps your skin to move toxins to the exterior and can be done either through exercise or steam bath or sauna. Take Epsom salt baths to draw toxins through the skin. If it is right, you may choose to use quarterly fasting to help your body detoxify. Hyperthermia cocoon heat therapy raises the core body temperature with dry heat and infrared to rid deep cells of waste products. Do colonic irrigation therapy to remove debris from your gut if needed.

#12 Accumulate Your Personal Armory

We all have our usual maladies to which we may succumb. We have our weaknesses. Yours may be catching viruses because of the grade school classroom you work in, or it could be painful joints due to a previous football injury. It could be digestive upset if your diet isn't exactly right, or even if it is. It could be sadness or anxiety due to life circumstances. It could be kidney stones, or a lower back disc herniation that is mostly under control, until it isn't. Have at the ready supplements, essential oils, infrared or laser therapy, moist heat packs, ice packs, and homeopathic remedies. Know a few trigger points for muscles spasm and pain relief,[111] and a few acupuncture points too. Every remedy we have and use is one less influence The System has over us. Use these tools, learn from others, and teach others.

Follow up on my resources page at *www.DrNancyTrimboli.com* and use your own new resources and books. Share with us on our *Trimboli Insiders Group* on Facebook. If you forget or need help, ask a question there. Especially important is to create an armory of immune boosters and germ fighters at home. Have at the ready: echinacea, essential oil blends, tea tree essential oil, olive leaf extract, colloidal silver, grapefruit seed extract, red marine algae, vitamin C, and vitamin D.

---

111 Trimboli, Nancy. Playlist: "Trigger Point Therapy," *YouTube*. Online videos - multiple. www.youtube/drnancytrimboli.com.

Forced at First

Linda, a retired librarian, usually consulted her conventional medical doctor for her health issues. She had a rough time over the last few years with pancreatic tumors, a knee replacement, and the loss of her husband from a terrible illness. She had a skin rash on both forearms, on and off for months. It was itchy, red and irritated, with small pustules. Was it a sudden new allergy to her cat? Certainly, she had a weakness due to the cancer treatment, and there was the severe emotional stress due to her loss of her husband. Was it all those things combined, or just one that may have caused it?

She had consulted a dermatologist who gave her a lengthy diagnosis, and her family physician, both of whom only recommended anti-inflammatory medication and cortisone lotion. After being on the drugs for months, her stomach was starting to bother her, that being a side effect of the medication. The skin rash continued to return.

Frustrated and at a dead-end, she started asking better questions. At first, it was forced. "*What if I could heal?*" she would say, even out loud with no one around, except the cat, to hear. It not only sounded forced, it felt that way too. She recalled hearing about colloidal silver from her friend, Alma who had used it for a toe fungus. Because Linda had used it previously, there was a spray bottle of it in her cabinet. She used it. "*It couldn't hurt,*" she thought. In four days, the rash was gone. Colloidal silver now has a place in her armory.

There is a world of opportunity for health and healing, and it's there waiting for you. It's in your town. It's in your memory. Your friend, maybe not named Alma, is part of it. It is also at our fingertips as the internet. Find it. Go to *www.DrNancyTrimboli.com* to discover resources now.

Start new healing routines. Make the time in your schedule. Demand that your self-care comes first. Only in that way can you take care of everyone else. Put yourself at the top of the Mission You priority list. Make me proud.

Mission You: Take Action

- For information and strategies to help you free yourself of The System, see www.DrNancyTrimboli.com for my favorite resources, and online courses.

- Share your new daily habits with our *Trimboli Insiders Group* on Facebook.

- Share your favorite components of your armory and see what is working for others.

- Let us know your triumphs!

Twelve Ways to Escape The System Checklist

- Clear time in your calendar for your own personal wellness.

- Surround yourself with supportive people.

- Be an example to others. They need help too.

- Get adjusted by a chiropractor monthly (or more if recommended.)

- Use massage therapy monthly (or more if recommended.)

- See an acupuncturist or energy medicine practitioner regularly.

- Eat clean.

- Count (and drink) your daily ounces of water.

- Sleep right.

- Exercise right.

- Detoxify.

- Assemble your own armory of supplements, methods, and other helpful things.

Chapter 8

THE NEW YOU

"Now ... I feel *joyous,*" Margaret said. "I've never felt joy in my life; not for years anyway. Not since I was ten or twelve years old. As an adult, I never knew what that was ... *joy.* I thought I was happy, but now I have true happiness that's part of me and not a response to something outside of me."

Margaret had been a patient of mine for six months. Her injury occurred while she was coaching her son's soccer team. It was a fluke injury to her foot. She had her foot on a soccer ball rolling it back to challenge the players. One of the boys ran up, stumbled, and his foot landed on top of Margaret's. The result was a fractured big toe, a small ligament tear, and a diagnosis of complex regional pain syndrome. After three months of physical therapy, she was still unable to work or drive and had to rely on family and friends to take her to my office. When I met her, she could not put any weight on the right foot or walk without the podiatry boot.

But changes were happening. At her one-month progress exam, she was the predicted 50% better, after three months 70% better. After six months, she was driving and able to describe the experience of her metamorphosis.

"Every morning, now, I am excited to get out of bed. I have goals, and I'm meeting them. I am organized. My kids aren't bored anymore. They have chores and a routine that is structured. A disciplined house is what they're flourishing on. They make better food choices; choosing an apple for a snack instead of something else. That's because *I'm* making better choices."

"God taught me a lesson with my injury. I came to a realization that conventional medical care had no place for healing. There was no progress. And now, with my chiropractic care I feel a transformation. I realize that I want to teach people about true purpose. That's what I want to do with my life. People need to know that when they feel stuck, it's because they have veered off the path of their purpose."

Margaret continued, "Everyone in my life is changing; even my husband and my mom. My friends, they say, 'Oh, my gosh. This is incredible. Can I get injured too?' What they meant is that they wanted to transform. 'Please don't take my path,' I told them. Don't wish yourself to get injured; a transformation takes just a moment. It's a decision, like flipping a light switch."

Margaret had been an RN for sixteen years. She didn't know how burned out she was until she was forced to stop working because of her injury. At her job, she noticed that some patients, once they reached the point where they were hospitalized for their conditions, would rarely become better. They'd be back in the hospital. Those were the regulars.

"It was sad," Margaret said, "because everyone has a choice in life, and these people made bad decisions, and they ended up back where they started. Granted, there would be those that would turn things around and get better. Some would die."

"My life had always been about *go, go, go, do, do, do*, but nothing ever really got done. There was never a feeling of peace. It was all done halfway. From stuffing food in my mouth in five minutes flat, to being so distracted that my kids never felt like I was ever there for them, not ever listening. I never exercised because I *thought* I was healthy. Reading wasn't part of my day. Honestly, I didn't have an identity. I didn't know who I was, because with little kids, you just survive each day. I felt lost. As my kids started to get older, my first thought was, *Maybe I should have another baby*. It never occurred to me to start to discover myself."

Margaret continues, "One evening, a while back, I was in the bathtub, wondering if I should file for an additional extension for my medical leave from work. I felt a sense of anxiety rise. A thought came to me, *What do I not want to be doing right now?* That was the turning point for me. I realized that my body, my intuition, was telling me something. That message from my intuition had been nagging me for a long time. I hadn't ever listened to it. My foot injury is what stopped me in my tracks. Quite literally. I couldn't walk, couldn't drive myself, I couldn't even stand. But it was only by stopping that I became more productive."

"I had time to reflect. My time in nursing was a necessary stage for me, and at the same time I knew there were bigger things in store. So, I watched videos on personal excellence, and the habits of successful people. *I want to be a successful person!* I thought. I started to read books on spirituality, on listening to your intuition, listening to your body, about organization and about living an exceptional life. These books talked about the impact you are making on other people's lives. I read and watched and read and watched."

"That day that I asked that question in my bathtub was after I had been under chiropractic care for a few weeks. I was finally feeling hopeful. I could see improvement. And the answer to that question was, *What I don't want to do is I don't want to be in that medical environment.* I had been an RN for sixteen years. I did that job because, well, that's what I was supposed to be doing. I never asked the question. I never asked, *Why do I wake up in a panic on the days I'm supposed to go to work?* My body had been telling me for years that I needed to get out of that environment. It was toxic for me. The sick just keep getting sicker. We could repair them temporarily, but they would be back due to the consequences of their own actions. For some, there's nothing to save them. It's like a boiled egg. You can't unboil it."

"It's after I asked the question, *What do I not want to do?* that I answered it. I didn't want to go to work there any longer. I decided, right there in the tub, that my time being an RN was over. The panic that I had felt when waking on my workdays would be done. I no longer had to worry over which patients would make poor choices and get sicker, or worse die, on my watch. In the next few days I realized there was another reason for my heart to be racing. It was *excitement.* I was now excited about life. All the reading and watching I was doing had given me a zest for living. I now had purpose."

"I am changing the lives of those around me. They ask me what I'm doing, and I share with them. If I could shout from the rooftops one thing that every human should do, especially if they would actually do it, I would tell them to put their own well-being first. You can't care for those you love unless you yourself are whole and healthy and energized. Put yourself first."

Margaret started where you may be right now. She was following the norms of The System because she didn't know what else to do. She had not even considered that other possibilities exist. Now she knows there is a world of opportunity, like you do. By quietly listening to her inner voice, she came to know her true purpose. It's a different path than what she has known her whole life. And she didn't have to travel far and wide to find it. It was within her all along. The changes she is making in herself are the catalyst of an evolution occurring with everyone around her. That is what is waiting for you. The number of people who know there is a better way toward health is surging, and you are part of it. Who knows … maybe one day, like Margaret, you'll be working on a book to help people transform and find *their* inner peace, joy, and happiness. "We are all human beings capable of something greater. It's in us and waiting to be found."

Margaret is not alone. These transformations happen every day. I've seen it in my office for years. As your body is cleared of interferences, toxins, and imbalances through holistic methods, it wakes up. You become more alive. It is happening to you right now. Because you have read this book, you have taken the first step. You are on a quest. You are asking better questions. As you heal and grow and learn, there is an evolution taking place. Naturally you are making better choices, noticing new options. You are more beautiful, with a brighter light in your eyes, are more charming and more attractive.

People see the change in you, and they want what you have. Teach them. Tell others what you have done. Share with them. They need to know. Imagine Margaret going through her life as she was; not "being there" with her kids, disregarding her body's calls for change, letting the timebomb tick, tick, tick away. Where would she be now? Where are *you* right now? Her life was transformed with seeking answers from better questions. You are asking better questions. Therein lies the brilliance. Take back your power. Resources and unexpected discoveries will be revealed. Stay on Mission You and unravel the mystery of you. Joy awaits.

Mission You doesn't end here. From years of being within the influences of The System, you have layers of injury, trauma, and stress to heal. But you are now resourceful and looking for answers. New opportunities will open up for you. Do not fear. Help is within reach. You are not alone. You have allies. Resources, like me, happily work outside of The System. Other undercover agents remain within The System but will help you to escape it.

Having your allies close and seeing your foes for who they are keeps you in control of your health. Knowing that there are avenues for true healing gives you confidence that help is always available.

The System is deviously powerful and is forever trying to draw you back, trying to trip you up. Advertising, your insurance coverage, conventional medical routines, your unenlightened friends and family, the food industry, the media, the chemical industry, many lawmakers and lobbyists are all part of The System. You cannot escape it. The difference is that now you are savvy to its efforts to disrupt your momentum.

Find comfort in knowing that the hard part is over. The realization that you have been duped is the biggest hurdle. I realize this is upsetting. But you didn't know. Let that be fuel to your fire and spread the word to others about what you have learned. And now, having read this book, a whole new world has opened up for you.

You are forever changed. Continue to return to your resources. Continue to learn. Share with others your discoveries, successes, and insights. Pace yourself and be patient with the process. Allow your body the time it needs to heal.

There is a surge of consciousness that will overcome The System. You are part of that change. But don't make a show of it…. Stealth is on our side.

In my early days in practice, I bought a wall sculpture from a local artist. It is a figure of a person expanding, almost dancing, out of a picture frame. It reminded me of the people I saw in my office who were experiencing chiropractic care. I was privileged to witness people emerge, just as in the sculpture. With their newly restored vitality they busted out of the confines of the bad stories they told themselves, away from fears produced by the media and conventional medicine and distanced themselves from the sickness created by poor choices and The System. Once they started chiropractic care, without trying, they made other healing changes in their lives. They ate better, quit jobs that were sapping their energy, returned to exercise. This is now you. You have inspired me, and I am proud of you for taking on this challenge. You have emerged from outdated thinking and habits that were restricting your ability to heal, to live, to love, and to learn. My hope is that the transition you have made is just the beginning of a permanent shift in perception of your own inborn miracle. Be well.

Acknowledgments

There is no way that I would be able to have put forth the time, mental energy, and effort to create this book without many of the people in my past and current life. The employees and staff of Trimboli Chiropractic over the years allowed me to do that of which I am most skilled: to teach a new way of healing and to deliver the chiropractic adjustment. You helped me to build a thriving large practice and to help many people emerge from helplessness to hope.

To my current staff for being one hundred percent behind my vision and me: I am eternally grateful for the care that you show to our patients and me. The extreme enthusiasm you exhibit is contagious. Thank you to Shelby, Jess, Marija, Daniel, Mary Ann, Melanie, Diana, Katie, and Missy. Sam, master of video creation, showed me a talent I didn't know I had.

To Anjanette Harper who took thirty-thousand words of cranky drivel and coaxed it into a fifty-three-thousand-word motivating, life-changing treatise for the most important individual I know, you the reader. Her one-on-one coaching, the content she created for her Top Three Book Workshop, and the authors and people with whom she surrounded me in the class were valuable beyond words.

A deep thanks to Jim C. for your generous help in the final, grueling edits. You made simple changes that reached out to my readers at an even deeper level. As A.J. Harper said, "Kudos. Good work."

To Dr. Sabrina Starling and the Tap the Potential team, all of my friends at the Breakthroughs on the Bayou retreat and in my small group (Todd, Jake, and Don) you have been more supportive to me and can convey the potential you see in me better than any other humans.

Thank you to my beta readers, your insights allowed me to polish this book and help me to see things that I was missing. To those whose stories came to me at the perfect moment: D.D., D.K., S.K., P.G., C.H., S.K., J.M., B.M., R.R., M.H., P.S., G.M., E.M. and to everyone that shared their stories, their vulnerabilities, and their yearnings for solutions: you inspire me.

To all of my patients: Thank you for allowing me to fulfill *my* life's purpose—To see the transformation in you so that you may experience the life you have dreamed of living.

For George, my husband of 25 years, who has been the rock that anchors my life which allows me to create and thrive, and just wants to spend time with me... *I'm back.*

About the Author

Dr. Nancy Trimboli is a health expert and chiropractor with over 25 years of experience. She has taken the lessons she learned from her father, an Episcopalian priest, and from earning a black belt in Taekwondo and used those as the foundation for her compassionate care of patients and for the hard work and dedication necessary to build a thriving business.

While in the heyday of her practice, Dr. Nancy created a multi-location, multi-doctor business with over 40 employees and she personally worked with up to 150 individual patients per day. This has allowed her to master the art of taking complex health issues and breaking them down into a concise and easy to comprehend manner. Dr. Nancy has facilitated over 800 workshops at her office. She shares her knowledge through platforms such as her YouTube channel (which currently has over 100 videos), Facebook live videos, and *Stealth Health: Take Back Your Power and Unravel the Mystery of You*, her first adult book. Her first children's book, *Little Squirrel Girl*, is a true story of a baby squirrel who needed a chiropractic adjustment and watched sunsets.

Index

CranioSacral therapy, 35, 38, 116, 149

cystitis, 32

D

desynchronosis, 132

direct-to-consumer-advertising (DTCA), 17

dizziness, 18, 44, 59

E

ear infection, 73, 88-89, 93

energy medicine practitioner, 38, 49, 77, 156

Ethan Hawke - *Mission Impossible*, 41-42, 51

evidence-based medicine, 35

F

Federal Trade Commission, 8-9, 24

Feldenkrais practitioner, 115

Food and Drug Administration, 8-9, 24

The Four Medical Testing Questions, 84, 91

functional medicine doctor, 65, 77, 86, 115, 147

G

G.A.P.S. diet book by Dr. Natasha Campbell-McBride, 75

gastritis, 36, 64

Gentempo, Patrick, 136

Graham, David, 25

H

headaches, 9, 27, 44, 87

heart attack, 21-24, 29, 57-59, 99

holosync, 38

homeopath, 6, 34, 38, 77, 87, 95, 96-98, 102, 104, 114, 127, 130, 137, 154

hypochlorhydria, 66-67, 69

I

Irritable Bowel Syndrome (IBS), 12, 51, 120

J
Jason Bourne - *Bourne Identity*, 52-53, 81, 110, 142-143

K
Kent, Christopher, 136
kidney failure, 3

L
lupus, 44-45
Lyme disease, 102-104, 137
Loudon, Mannette, 25

M
male infertility, 4
May, Katy, 27-28
Medicare, 3
Mercola.com, 26, 75
midwife, 8
Mission You, 8-10, 13-14, 20, 36-37, 39-40, 42, 46, 48-49, 51, 53-55, 59, 62-64, 67, 69, 73, 78-79, 81-83, 86, 88, 90-91, 93, 110-111, 113, 116, 119, 122-123, 130, 138-139, 143-144, 146, 151, 155-156, 160
Mission You Journal Pages, 55, 79
multiple sclerosis (MS), 109
Murray, Michael and Joseph Pizzorno - *Encyclopedia of Natural Medicine*, 66, 69, 122
My Healthcare Arsenal, 55, 79, 123, 139
My Key Motivators, 40
Myofascial Release, 38, 149

N
NAET (Nambudripad's Allergy Elimination Technique), 74

O

P

R

S

T